The International Behavioural and Social Sciences Library

SIX MINUTES FOR THE PATIENT

T0386364

TAVISTOCK

The International Behavioural and Social Sciences Library

HEALTH & SOCIETY
In 12 Volumes

SIX MINUTES FOR THE PATIENT

Interactions in General Practice Consultation

EDITED BY ENID BALINT
AND J S NORELL

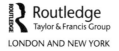

LONDON AND NEW YORK

First published in 1973 by
Tavistock Publications Limited

Published in 2001 by
Routledge
2 Park Square, Milton Park, Abingdon, Oxfordshire OX14 4RN
711 Third Avenue, New York, NY 10017

First issued in paperback 2014

Routledge is an imprint of the Taylor and Francis Group, an informa business

British Library Cataloguing in Publication Data
A CIP catalogue record for this book
is available from the British Library

Six Minutes for the Patient
ISBN 0-415-26424-3
Health & Society: 12 Volumes
ISBN 0-415-26509-6
The International Behavioural and Social Sciences Library
112 Volumes
ISBN 0-415-25670-4

ISBN 13: 978-1-138-88136-5 (pbk)
ISBN 13: 978-0-415-26424-2 (hbk)

Six Minutes
for the Patient

INTERACTIONS IN GENERAL
PRACTICE CONSULTATION

Edited by
ENID BALINT &
J. S. NORELL

TAVISTOCK PUBLICATIONS

First published in 1973
by Tavistock Publications Limited
2 Park Square, Milton Park, Abingdon, Oxon, OX14 4RN

ISBN 0 422 74270 8

Distributed in the U.S.A. by
HARPER & ROW PUBLISHERS, INC.
BARNES & NOBLE IMPORT DIVISION

Contents

Editors' Foreword

The research on which this book is based was carried out between 1966 and 1971 on case-reports submitted by the following general practitioners, who were members of the group:

Dr H. J. Carne   Dr A. J. Hawes (until 1968)
Dr M. B. Clyne   Dr P. Hopkins
Dr M. J. F. Courtenay   Dr A. Lask
Dr J. Foster (until 1967)   Dr J. S. Norell
Dr C. H. Gill   Dr H. S. Pasmore

The reports were presented at weekly seminars held, under the leadership of the Balints, at the Department of Psychological Medicine, University College Hospital, London. The following psychiatrists attended as associates, and contributed to the discussions:

Dr H. A. Bacal (from 1970–1971)
Dr Mary L. Hare
Dr C. P. Treves-Brown

In addition many colleagues, some of them from abroad, visited our group on one or more occasions, and our thanks are due to all of them for their helpful contributions.

We are especially grateful to the late Dr E. W. Dunkley and to Dr R. F. Tredgold who kindly put rooms at our disposal in their department for our seminars, and who continued to take a close interest in the progress of our work; to the principal secretary of the Department, Miss Jean Mann; to Mrs Monica Howes and Mrs Dorothy Hone who transcribed the recorded discussions and produced a verbatim account from often unpromising material; and to Dr Mary Hare, who devoted a great deal of time to reading the draft chapters and making very many valuable suggestions, and corrected the proofs.

Nor have we overlooked the patients themselves, whose records form the raw material of our study. We have been concerned to ensure that none of them should be recognized, except, possibly, by themselves, and to this end we have taken the following steps:

(i) The patients' names have been altered.

(ii) Their doctors have been given pseudonyms.

(iii) Place names, which might identify the location of practices, have also been changed.

These alterations are constant throughout the text and the reader will still be able to follow a particular case, comparing aspects of it treated in the different chapters.

Michael Balint led the seminars jointly with Enid Balint until his death in December 1970. During the five years of his co-leadership he scarcely missed a single meeting of the thirty or so held each year. He led the group with energy, humour and understanding. We should like to think that these qualities are reflected in this book (which had been only partly drafted at the time of his death) and that the work as a whole bears the stamp of freshness of outlook and sceptical scrutiny which Michael Balint inspired in us and for which he was renowned.

London,   *Enid Balint*
June 1972.   *J. S. Norell*

Introduction

J. S NORELL

. . . the occasion when, in the intimacy of the consulting room,
a person who is ill, or believes himself to be ill, seeks the advice of
a doctor whom he trusts. This is a consultation . . .

Sir James Spence

The patient brings his symptoms; the doctor prescribes a remedy
or gives advice. What really happens during such consultations in
general practice? In the short time they are together (six minutes on
the average) what is the doctor able to learn about his patient, and
what has the patient been able to convey about himself? What can
be achieved during such fleeting episodes?

These are a few of the questions that come to mind as one
ponders the mystery of the general practice consultation. Similar
questions intrigued Michael and Enid Balint who already had
unrivalled insight into the nature of general practice. Eager for
more understanding in this area they set out in 1966 together with a
group of seasoned general practitioners on yet another exploration.
This book is a record of that experience.

Six years were spent on the study of this six-minute interview.
Here, we report at length on such questions as the research
methodology and its validation, and on the strategy and tactics of
the interview. Nonetheless, our work is firmly rooted in everyday
general practice; this book is first and foremost an account of the
ordinary consultation, the sort in which general practitioners are
engaged thirty or forty times each working day. This is what we
were looking at—or it might be truer to say looking down on
initially. For to some of us general practitioners it appeared

improbable that the trivia of our daily work could be worth spending time studying or would stand up to critical examination. It was with some scepticism therefore that we joined the search for the gems which Michael Balint had always insisted were there in general practice, waiting to be discovered.

We did find something (though not exactly what we had been expecting) and as a result we general practitioners in the group began to see our routine work in a fresh light. Formerly, thanks to values inculcated by early hospital training, general practice had been regarded as concerned merely with sorting occasional grains of wheat from the predominant chaff, a philosophy which led many doctors to seek their professional satisfaction in the picking up of 'worthwhile' cases from relatively unpromising material. That attitude had already come under fire from Balint in 1957, and receives a further broadside as a result of the present study.

The renaissance in general practice, a phenomenon of the 1960's, owed a great deal to the recognition of the enormous therapeutic potential in the doctor/patient relationship, a factor to which Balint had opened the eyes of the profession and which he had begun to examine scientifically. His influence went far beyond the handful of doctors who were privileged to work with him, and is to be found now in every area of general practice. We hope the description of this research, and the arguments derived from its results, will help to put this approach to general practice on an even firmer footing.

Before passing on to a brief account of the individual chapters, a word about the general arrangement. It may be regarded as falling into two main sections, clinical and technical. Following Michael Balint's exposition of the research come three chapters principally concerned with the clinical process itself: what is going on during the face to face contact. The authors examine the consultation from different standpoints and describe the various techniques we discovered were being employed in the interviews. The more technical section starts with a description of the Form used to collate our data. Succeeding chapters examine such topics as diagnosis, predictions, the follow-up, research methodology, the time element, and the sharing of patients with specialist colleagues. The concluding chapter, by Enid Balint, looks back over the research, and forward too, for as well as answering some questions our work has thrown up fresh ones.

In his chapter, 'Research in Psychotherapy', Michael Balint traces the origins of the current research back to some of his previous ventures. The point of departure for the present study was the realization that the psychotherapeutic techniques then in use in general practice were of very limited application in the doctor's day-to-day work. A few patients would be selected for special interviews and as a consequence the doctor's work became split into fairly watertight compartments. The selection, though rationalized by the doctor, was felt by him to be unsatisfactory and remained a source of irritation.

The aim of the present research was to explore the application of psychotherapeutic techniques to ordinary general practice. This was done by looking at apparently successful examples of such work, chosen by the doctors themselves, which had been accomplished during normal consultations. The majority of these consultations had lasted from five to fifteen minutes. Those longer than average were acceptable for the research, provided that consultations of such length were normally accommodated in the consulting session of the doctor concerned. Balint reviews the development of the research, illustrating his points with a detailed discussion of one of the case-reports.

With Enid Balint's chapter, 'The Flash Technique', we are immediately plunged into a debate on what it is that should be aimed for in the general practice consultation. She argues that the traditional aim of pinpointing the seat of the trouble may not always be appropriate. An alternative aim would be to provide the patient with the opportunity to communicate whatever it is he wants, and this can result in a brief, intense and close contact. Any problems that are exposed by this 'flash' can be explored in subsequent interviews, but in such exploration the patient uses the doctor: to a great extent the patient himself determines the pace and content of the work they do together. The essence of the particular kind of work which Enid Balint describes is that the doctor tries to focus his attention on what it is the patient is trying to convey at that particular time, rather than on the underlying causes, though of course the latter may engage his attention on subsequent occasions.

At this point in the argument, doctors might well feel some uneasiness because they have much less to guide them in this way of working than with the more traditional approach. Theories exist, for example, on the long-term effects of emotional deprivation in early childhood, but what theories are there about the present—and therefore unique—interaction which is taking place between doctor and patient? Undeterred, Enid Balint would have doctors abandon—or, as she sees it, be liberated from—their theories in such cases. The doctor who is preoccupied with theories may fail to notice, or to recall, or to utilise for therapy, quite ordinary but significant events in the consultation. He may instead pursue questions which are really side-issues of the patient's present problem, but which seem to fit in better with the doctor's own constructs.

A case-report illustrates these ideas and highlights the difficulty found in sustaining sufficiently attentive observation. This in turn leads to a discussion of the problem of the proper exploitation of the flash. It appears however that the successful application of the 'tuning-in' technique enables the doctor to achieve some understanding of what the patient really wants of him, and this can be accomplished without paying the price of a too-dependent and clinging relationship.

'The Patient's Use of his Doctor' is the theme taken up by Stephen Pasmore. He recalls how, having acquired an 'apostolic function' (from a proficiency in 'doing psychotherapy'), we doctors were then reluctant to abandon the role of the detective in charge of the investigations. Until we did so, however, we were unable to get in touch with our patients in the ordinary consultation, in a properly therapeutic way. Pasmore quotes, by way of a cautionary tale, a case-report showing how the doctor's traditional technique, while it resulted in a good overall diagnosis, brought him no nearer an understanding of what was wanted of him at that particular moment. Doctor and patient were in effect at cross-purposes: he wanting to get at the cause of her anxieties, she needing him as some kind of support for her defences. By attempting to fit his

xii

observations into categories that he had already understood the doctor remained insensitive to aspects of the communication to which, had he been 'tuned-in', he might have been able to respond more therapeutically.

The contrasts in the different approaches to the consultation are further analysed by Cyril Gill in his chapter, 'Types of Interview in General Practice'. He describes three consecutive consultations with one patient, a middle-aged spinster who felt tired and sluggish. Each interview, it transpired, employed a different technique and had a different outcome. The first consultation, clearly illness-orientated, was dominated by the doctor's efforts to identify an illness, in this case myxoedema or anaemia. The second consultation was patient-orientated and the doctor learned a good deal about his patient, in particular of her sense of isolation, but did not engage her feelings. He did accomplish this in the third interview, by making use of a new awareness about the patient. His response to the flash at once put the relationship on to a different footing and enabled the patient to see more of herself, particularly the way she related to other people.

The illumination of significant new areas can transform the situation, allowing doctor and patient to cut across the mass of biographical data conventionally regarded as a *sine qua non* of any psychodynamic formulation. As Gill points out, the usual pattern of doctor/patient contacts in general practice is an extended one. Where contacts are so episodic, fleeting and apparently disconnected, it is the flash technique which holds promise for effective intervention.

A good deal of time was spent in the seminars discussing how best to record the observations the doctors brought. It had always been customary in Balint Seminars to allow the doctor to tell his story in his own way, much as we should allow a patient to do. This often meant that the account lacked an orderly presentation: there were apparent contradictions, back-tracking, hesitations, blurting out of information. But the ensuing confusion was acceptable because something of value emerged which probably could not have been achieved in any other way.

First of all we became familiar with the reporting doctor's individual style and his approach to his work. We came to know whether he was diffident or brash; the sort of cases he felt at home with, and the ones he tended to avoid. Over a course of time he gave us a standard of what was normal for him which we could apply to his subsequent case-reports. Then, against this background, his behaviour within the group would be found time and time again to reflect the doctor/patient contact in the consulting room. When in his seminars Balint departed from the tradition of 'bedside' teaching, he did so in the secure knowledge that the absence of the patient himself was no loss: the central subject of study, the doctor/patient relationship, was present, mirrored in the group/ doctor interaction. Free from the constraints of a formal and logical presentation the reporting doctor was able to represent—almost to impersonate—his patient. In this way the group was vouchsafed a glimpse of what truly went on in the consulting room.

When we began our research into the ordinary consultation we realized we should require specific information, uniformly presented, covering a large number of areas. The reporting doctor might eventually have revealed much of this but we needed a system which could be relied on to catch potentially important ideas which the work might throw up, and into which could be fed data in an identifiable form, gathered in a uniform way. In his chapter, 'The Development of the Form' Michael Courtenay describes our attempts to solve this problem. By means of a case-report he traces the development of the initial and follow-up Forms (reproduced in Appendix 'A') and shows how each new concept would be reflected in the adoption of fresh headings, while ideas that had led us into cul-de-sacs were gradually abandoned.

A medical aphorism declares that treatment must be preceded by diagnosis. But what sort of diagnosis? Of skin disorders it was held, perhaps cynically, that diagnosis lay between the conditions which responded and those which did not respond to calamine lotion. (This was before the advent of cortico-steroids!) To a great extent however, the sort of diagnosis we make in general practice reflects the range of treatment available. Is this true for the psychotherapeutic aspects of general practice?

Introduction

This is the question to which Max Clyne addresses himself in the chapter, 'The Diagnosis'. He discussses what the function of a diagnosis should be and contrasts the traditional with the overall diagnosis. The former categorizes the illness so that what is known of its natural history shall indicate the outlook for the patient and be a guide to rational treatment. It has the additional function, Clyne points out, of lessening anxiety, for by naming the illness we appear to be removing it from the realm of the unknown. The traditional diagnosis is illness-centred.

The shortcomings in this approach, especially where emotional factors are prominent, are revealed in an extended case-report. The main criticism is that the traditional diagnosis has little or nothing to say about the person who is ill. Clyne gives examples of this and goes on to assess the value of the wider, patient-centred, overall diagnosis. If the latter were sufficiently comprehensive it would take account of those very features missing from traditional formulations: the external pressures on the patient, his internal world, his relationship with significant people around him, and, of great importance in this sort of work, the way in which the doctor/patient relationship has developed. With a case-report which spans three years Clyne shows that an overall diagnosis can indeed be valuable in directing the doctor's attention to those areas of the patient's life which require exploring. Further, it can provide a guide to the form the treatment should take if it is to be fully effective.

How is this to be accomplished in the course of ordinary general practice? This emerged as the central problem for the seminar. Under the stimulus of the research special efforts could be made and much useful information gathered, but in an ordinary consultation, even in a series of such consultations, the piecing together of a really comprehensive diagnosis would appear to be impracticable. An alternative possibility was the focal diagnosis entailing a narrowing down of the area of interest. Selective attention and its corollary, selective neglect, though part and parcel of clinical practice, had not previously been examined in a systematic way. The focal concept did not prove to be particularly appropriate to our sort of work and was soon abandoned by us. We eventually arrived at our present understanding: selection must occur, but it would be performed primarily by the patient. The focus would not be pre-selected by the doctor.

We had travelled back to another medical aphorism: 'Listen to the patient; he is telling you the diagnosis!'

How was the research to be validated, seeing that we could not mount a controlled trial of the drug, 'doctor'? In the chapter, 'On Predictions', Aaron Lask explains our approach to this problem: we compared predictions about a patient with the actual outcome. To do this properly entailed keeping to a discipline of accurate diagnostic formulations, precise treatment plans, and reliable follow-up reports. The adoption of this regime brought complications in its wake. For instance, the pursuit of more precision led to preoccupation with fine detail so that biographical data in the case assumed a disproportionate significance. Treatment plans were found to be at variance with what the doctor eventually did. (We later came to appreciate that the treatment plan was not to be regarded as a fixed quantity, any more than a diagnosis was, but capable of being continually modified in response to new understandings about the patient.) Then again, it was often impossible to determine whether the outcome was the result of the doctor's treatment, or, so to speak, spontaneous. Matters were not helped by the rather non-committal terms in which some of the predictions were stated. The vagueness was understandable since we were being asked for more than a general prognosis based on probabilities; the challenge to specify the course of future events was not fully met until we acquired the courage of our convictions.

A dilemma we found ourselves in was how to satisfy the research protocol without affecting the nature of the consultations we were observing. This problem is constantly being encountered in behavioural studies and to some extent in every scientific investigation. In the course of trying to resolve this we made some progress towards measuring the effectiveness of the doctor's treatment. Although his intervention might have a substantial impact, dubbed 'big bang', we found it could often be better understood in terms of an accumulation of 'little bangs'. We learned that in evaluating the progress of a patient it was necessary to pay attention not only to his symptomatology but to changes in the doctor/patient relationship, and to the tensions in the significant people around him. This led us to devise a system of scoring—the rating scales. (These rating scales,

xvi

together with a commentary by Howard Bacal, are reproduced in Appendix 'B').

Lask concludes that the limitations of time in the ordinary consultation, although imposing constraints, may actually operate in such a way as to promote the emergence of the flash. Convincing evidence of the effectiveness of the flash should come with more accurate predictions; meanwhile it relies on the feeling of work well done.

Assessing the effectiveness of treatment in patient-orientated medicine is the problem further considered by Howard Bacal in his chapter, 'Validation of the Research'. He lists a number of criteria by which the adequacy of a clinical trial may be judged and examines how well our research came up to these criteria. The inappropriatness of conventional control material led to our using the patient as his own control in a before-and-after comparison. The reporting doctor was asked to nominate one of the therapeutic options available to him and to make predictions based on this. This furnished us with a statement linking the four variables in the case: the patient, the illness, the doctor and the treatment. We had failed, however, to distinguish between two sets of objectives in the treatment: the work to be done in the therapy situation, and longer term goals which might be expected to follow as a result of successful therapy. Once this had been appreciated a framework was established in which treatment techniques could be studied.

On the question of the reliability of the ratings, an objective demonstration of this might have been achieved had the research been designed to allow for a panel of independent raters. We relied however on an internal assessment. Bacal emphasises that the criteria for the ratings had undergone many revisions, the scores allotted in each of the areas were arrived at by consensus, and that our own critical scrutiny of the case-reports led, if anything, to a playing down of our achievements.

A final point concerns the comparability of the conditions under which the research was conducted with the normal situation in the field. There were two special circumstances which must be taken into account when evaluating the research. First, the general practitioners in the group were already highly experienced in the

xvii

application of psychotherapeutic techniques to patients in general practice. Second, the leadership of the seminars undoubtedly contributed to the quality of the achievement. Our results, Bacal concludes, are true for this group of doctors led by this pair of analysts. How others would have fared, he leaves an open question.

When we came to review the scores that had been allotted under the various headings, certain patterns seemed to emerge. In a chapter on 'Follow-Ups' Aaron Lask examines these patterns to see whether they correlate with different types of case. He finds that some of the scoring patterns are characteristic. For instance, uniformly high scores were found in cases that went well, as might be expected. Others showed high scores for the doctor/patient relationship and low values in the other areas (patient's condition, tensions around the patient, work done), suggesting an element of collusion with the patient. Some cases showed the reverse of this picture, with the relationship scoring relatively low while other aspects appeared improved. Lask's explanation for this is that deterioration in the relationship led to the patient avoiding the doctor by a retreat into health.

Several cases had uniformly low scores, reflecting the situation in which nothing appeared to be happening for a considerable length of time. Whether this was due to the patient's innate resistance or for want of a better technique on the part of the doctor could not be decided from the material available. A negative score in one or more of the areas was taken to indicate a failure. In such cases it was often possible during the later group discussions to see what should have been done—or not done. But this was rarely due to new information coming to light. The doctor, it seemed, had been handicapped not by lack of information but by a kind of insensitivity to his patient's communication. The communication had been noted—it had been reported; but it had not been fully understood at the time. Lask believes that further familiarity with 'flash' work will enhance the doctor's sensitivity and will bring about a consistently better performance.

Next, Philip Hopkins tackles a vexed question in 'The Time Factor'. He contrasts the seemingly unlimited time for clinical

Introduction

procedures offered the student during his hospital teaching with the strictly limited time available—five or six minutes on the average —for consultations in general practice. Hopkins says that time of this order is sufficient only for making a spot diagnosis, or, in less straightforward cases, for deciding on a fairly obvious course of action such as referral to a specialist. For many, for perhaps the majority of patients whose illnesses reflect emotional disturbance, their problems cannot be properly resolved in either of these ways. Hopkins takes the NHS to task for not providing the conditions in which adequate time would be available to general practitioners for the proper investigation and treatment of all such patients.

The research-cum-training seminars run by Michael and Enid Balint offered the hope of adequately helping some at least of these patients in general practice, and the opportunity was eagerly seized by a few doctors who, in time, became adept at employing psychotherapeutic techniques in interviews lasting generally from thirty to sixty minutes. Balint is quoted as saying in 1957 that it was the doctor's responsibility to find time for long interviews whenever this was indicated, and that the plea of shortage of time might be fallacious. By 1966 however, the search was on for a way of using these techniques in the ordinary general practice consultation lasting from five to ten minutes; it had been appreciated that psychotherapeutic techniques, far from being integrated into general practice, had remained a 'foreign body', in constant danger of being extruded. One of the alternatives that was canvassed was a concentrated shortened version of the long interview. But just as Balint had insisted in his original training seminars, he was not offering 'watered-down psycho-analysis', so now too, there was no great enthusiasm for the 'mini-long-interview' as it was called.

When the 'flash' came to be recognized, its chief attraction for us was that it was not time-dependent, but intensity-dependent; that is, intensity of observation, of identification, and of communication. It offered a way of reaching the patient swiftly. In spite of this, Hopkins is sceptical about the long-term usefulness of the flash technique, though he concedes that it may have a place as a screening procedure. He finds that of the forty or so cases reported in the seminar, just under half were associated with a flash; and of these, just over half proceeded to longer interviews.

Hopkins quotes at length from the seminar discussions—one might almost say he gives chapter and verse—to support his reservations. (The extracts do vividly recall the way we wrestled with this problem.) He clearly disapproves of what he sees as revisionist movements which fail to keep true to Balint's original aims. Prominent amongst those indicated (this would have amused and delighted him) is Balint himself.

Some of the patients whose cases were reported at the seminars were receiving treatment in addition to that being provided by the reporting doctor. This second source proved most often to be either an orthopaedic surgeon or a psychotherapist. Michael Courtenay looks at these cases in a chapter entitled 'One Patient, Two Doctors'. This study, though peripheral to our main research interest, nevertheless raises issues clearly of great importance for the fuller understanding of the nature of general practice. Where two doctors are treating one patient there is ample opportunity for competitiveness, ambiguity, confusion over accountability, and doubt in regard to the cause of any improvement and the correct understanding of fresh developments in the illness.

At times the patient may be a victim of the confusion between his doctors. On the other hand he may be seen quite clearly exploiting, or even promoting, such confusion. On occasions the doctor may employ referral as a means of evading the implications of his over-all diagnosis. Courtenay makes the point forcibly that in the face of abdication by the general practitioner, specialist help will in itself prove of no avail so far as the central problem is concerned. But where specialist referral is appropriate, the doctor's continued and active responsibility for the case can increase the effectiveness of the patient's total care.

Winding up with a personal view of our work, Enid Balint, in the 'Epilogue', emphasises that, as she sees it, the research into the general practice consultation was undertaken not to find short cuts to the longer psychotherapeutic interview, but to measure as precisely as possible the therapeutic potential of the doctor/patient relationship in its everyday setting. Her chapter concludes our collective report, the imperfections in which must be freely acknowledged. The absence, in particular, of a sense of finality or even of a firm conclusion may strike the reader as somewhat odd, but this deficiency, if it really be one, is intentional. We were reporting, as Enid Balint reminds us, at a time when the work was on-going; this account was meant to be in the nature of a progress report to stimulate further studies, rather than a definitive statement. Moreover the way in which individual contributors have presented their own—and at times, idiosyncratic—views has itself been a valuable corrective against the assumption of authoritative postures. In this respect, as in many others, the book reflects the way we worked in the seminars.

It has been the purpose of this introduction to set out the book's principal themes: it cannot hope to convey more than a hint of the richness of the work itself. In the succeeding chapters these themes are fully developed by other members of the group. The extracts from our case discussions will especially help to bring the work alive for the reader who will discover in the following pages what first aroused our curiosity, inspired us to plan the research, sustained us through six years, and finally brought this study to fruition.

CHAPTER 1

Research in Psychotherapy[1]

MICHAEL BALINT

The research about which we are reporting started in January 1966 when the research team met for the first time. The ideas that led us to plan this research originated from two sources.

One source was our attempts at enabling doctors to recognize and understand their patients' complaints, not only in terms of illnesses, but also in terms of personal conflicts and problems, and then to use this understanding so that it should have a therapeutic effect. This research started in the autumn of 1950 and is still going on. In the first instance it meant introducing into medical practice something modelled on the techniques of an enlightened psychiatric interview. However, right from the start we recognized the differences between the psychiatric interview and the new technique that was needed in medical practice, and emphasized it by referring to the latter as 'listening' or 'long interview'; we also coined the phrase: 'he who asks questions will get answers—but hardly anything else'.

In spite of all the effort to create a technique suited to the setting of medical practice, the 'long interview' has remained a sort of foreign body in the general practitioner's normal routine. One of the many reasons why this had to be so is in fact its length. The average patient gets about ten to fifteen minutes from his doctor, while the 'long interview' needs about forty to fifty minutes. One of the unforeseen, and definitely undesirable, side-effects of this new technique was that from then on the doctor was forced to have two

[1] One version was read in Paris at the International Congress of the Société Française de Médecine Psychosomatique in September 1970 and published in the *Revue de Médecine Psychosomatique et de Psychologie Médicale*, No. 3, 1970.

1

classes of patients: with one class he persevered with the methods he had learned at his teaching hospital, which we called illness-centred medicine, while with the other class he practised patient-centred medicine based on long interviews.

The other source of our ideas was our study of the psychiatric interview and later of the techniques needed in short-term psychotherapy or psychotherapy with limited aims. These tasks were undertaken in the second half of the fifties, by a team consisting of trained psychoanalysts, which became known as the Workshop. In present-day psychiatric thinking, under the increasing influence of psychoanalytic ideas, the observations made in any sort of psychotherapy are described in the first instance in terms of psychopathology or psychodynamics. Both these sets of terms, in particular the latter, have become a sort of battle-cry; and one often hears phrases like dynamic psychotherapy or dynamically orientated psychotherapy.

In contrast to this way of thinking, we tried to concentrate our research on the study of the therapeutic processes. We soon had to learn that thinking in psychopathological or psychodynamic terms offered us only limited help for the understanding of these processes. Because every therapy is based on an interplay between patient and doctor, it cannot be really understood if one restricts one's observations either to the one or to the other: the therapy happens not in the patient nor in the doctor but between the two of them. If this is acceptable, it follows that what has to be observed and recorded is the interdependence or interaction between patient and doctor. This new approach brought fruitful results but proved rather difficult. Time and again we regressed to our old ways of observing and recording the events pertaining to one individual only; that is, we reverted to psychopathology or psychodynamics. To counteract this tendency in ourselves we devised forms for recording the results of our interviews. This proved to be a very hard discipline and practically all of us revolted at one time or another against it. It cost us hard work to recognize the need for this discipline and still more work to appreciate its value.

These forms have been ever since a most important tool in all subsequent researches. Chapter 5 will describe the history of these

2

forms in our present research, how they changed and developed with our increasing experience and insight. To show their spirit, here are a few samples of the headings, devised by our earliest research teams in the fifties, which have remained with us and become almost 'classical'. One heading runs: 'Development of the Interview' and then asks '(a) how patient treated doctor' and '(b) how doctor treated patient'. Another heading runs: 'Atmosphere of the Interview', and then specifies: '(a) patient's contributions' and '(b) therapist's contributions'. A third heading enquires about: 'Interpretations thought of and given' and contrasts them with 'Interpretations thought of but not given', and so on.

No matter how exactly the patient's psychopathology is known, it does not provide reliable enough material to answer any of these headings. I hope it will become evident that, in order to answer these headings adequately, a different sort of observation and a different way of thinking are needed. The work of the Workshop led to the discovery of a new method of psychotherapy which we called *focal therapy*.

In its fully developed form it enabled us to decide—fairly adequately—even in the diagnostic period what the therapist should aim at, approximately how many sessions he would need to achieve his aims, and what the approximate results of his therapy would be. The preconditions for a focal approach were: (a) that we could isolate in the patient's mind, using our observations in the first few interviews, a fairly well defined area, which we called the *focal area* or *focus*; (b) that we could see the possibility of helping the patient to a considerable readjustment in this area; and lastly (c) that this readjustment could lead to important improvements in the patient's whole life situation. In order to achieve all this in a limited number of sessions, a new technique was devised aiming at restricting the therapeutic work, as far as possible, to the focal area. The chief characteristics of this new technique were what we called *selective attention* and *selective neglect*. This meant that, whenever possible, the therapist should choose interpretations which lead the patient's associations towards the focal area and neglect others which might lead the work away from it. If the focal area was correctly chosen the patient's associations showed a marked trend towards the area; on the other hand, if this trend did not appear we

3

had to admit that our diagnosis was incorrect. In some cases choosing a new focal area led to the desired results; in others, the therapeutic work developed into a long-term therapy or proved unsuccessful.[2]

The demands made on the therapist by the focal technique are somewhat different from those made by psychoanalysis. The work hardly ever reaches far down into the pregenital regions; similarly the transference does not show many primitive pregenital characteristics; the therapy tends to remain on the whole object, i.e. genital level—in this way the therapist has an easier task. On the other hand he cannot relax to the form of free-floating attention, but must be always on the alert to choose—according to the principle of selective neglect and selective attention—how to respond to the patient's associations so that the work should be led towards the focal area and not away from it. This close interaction between therapist and patient is perhaps the most important factor that brings about the result of short-term therapy.

In our experience analysts are the best material for learning this new technique, but not all of them; some of them find its spirit so much against the principles of classical analytic technique that they cannot ever become familiar with it. On the other hand some non-analysed doctors or psychiatrists are able to acquire sufficient skills in this technique to enable them to do acceptable therapy.[3]

Since the beginning of the 1960's we have experimented with focal therapy techniques in various research seminars consisting of general practitioners. The results were fairly good, even encouraging, but one essential disadvantage remained unchanged: focal therapy, in the same way as the earlier 'listening during a long interview', remained a foreign body in the normal routine of medical practice. This meant that it remained impossible to offer therapy for every patient who in the doctor's opinion needed it. The doctor was thus forced to select and treat some of his patients, in

---

[2] For a more detailed description see Malan (1963). A detailed follow-up study of *all* the cases treated by the members of the Workshop is in preparation.

[3] See, for instance, Max B. Clyne: *Night Calls*; L. J. Freedman: *Virgin Wives*; R. S. Greco: *One Man's Practice*; A. Lask: *Asthma*; M. J. F. Courtenay: *Sexual Discord in Marriage*, etc., all in the Mind and Medicine Monographs, Tavistock Publications 1962-1969.

fact the majority, by the methods of illness-centred medicine and only a few with the new techniques of patient-centred medicine.

By 1965 the two of us, Enid Balint and I, had to realize that the techniques deriving from the idea of focal therapy were not the answer to this important problem. They certainly eased the pressure on the practitioner but they could not be used as part of his normal routine. In consequence, we decided to organize a research team to find out whether new techniques could be designed which would enable the doctor to offer psychological help to any of his patients without disrupting the normal routine of his practice. We excluded from our investigation any form of non-specific, and therefore questionable, method such as: general support, wholesale reassurance, well-meant sympathetic advice, and any sort of watered-down psychoanalysis. The new techniques that we were aiming at had to be based on a reliable understanding of the patient's individuality and of the developing relationship between patient and doctor, on the one hand, and on the other it should be possible for a large enough proportion of doctors to acquire sufficient skill in them without previous personal analysis; and lastly, the time needed for these techniques should be compatible with the routine ten to fifteen minutes that the average patient gets in a medical practice. It was this last condition that led to the name of 'ten-minute psychotherapy'.

We anticipated that our research would encounter serious difficulties so we decided to invite to our team only a few well-experienced colleagues, all of whom had participated for several years in our seminars. In this way this seminar, UCH/4, is fundamentally different from any previous ones: its members are not spontaneous volunteers, but, one could almost say, invited conscripts. In spite of it, the team proved very constant; in the four-and-a-half years[4] of our existence we lost only two of the original nine. One of our members had to withdraw because his hearing deteriorated so that he found working in a group impossible, and only one had to withdraw because of his disappointment. In the second year of our existence an experienced colleague asked to be

[4] This chapter was written by Michael Balint before he died in December, 1970; the work of the seminar continued until July, 1972.

admitted to the research team. It was these eight doctors, H. J. Carne, M. B. Clyne, M. J. F. Courtenay, C. H. Gill, P. Hopkins, A. Lask, J. S. Norell and H. S. Pasmore, on whose clinical work this research has been based. Our work gradually attracted interest and we were joined first by two psychiatrists, both experienced psychotherapists, Dr Mary L. Hare and Dr C. P. Treves-Brown, and lately by Dr H. A. Bacal, a fully trained psychoanalyst. Right at the start the team accepted the condition that every patient reported was to remain a research case and had to be followed up automatically at regular intervals of ten to eighteen months. At the end of his initial report the doctor was asked to state explicitly what his therapeutic plans were and what he expected to achieve with them. As all our transactions were recorded and then transcribed, at the follow-up period it was easy to decide whether or not the predictions were correct, i.e. whether the therapy decided upon and administered was effective or not. Perhaps it ought to be mentioned that these conditions are more stringent than those generally used for testing the efficiency of any psychotherapeutic method, including the psychoanalytic one.

Since at the start we had no idea, only hopes, whether anything like our expectation was feasible at all, we asked the doctors to report any interview during which they thought that they had succeeded in making a meaningful contact with the patient and, using this, they had achieved something acceptable, provided that the interview did not last longer than ten to fifteen minutes.

The team started off with great enthusiasm, which was fostered by a fair number of cases which seemed to prove that it is possible, even under these strict conditions, to understand the patient reliably and to use this understanding so that it should have a therapeutic effect. Soon we encountered serious difficulties when we tried to define more exactly what sort of observations were needed in the follow-up period to validate or refute reliably the predictions made in the initial period. What we learned in this way made us re-examine the reliability of our therapeutic techniques initially accepted. This led to a crisis in our research. Everything had to be challenged and some of the doctors became so discouraged that there was serious danger that the research might have to be abandoned. Eventually the team was able to diagnose the causes of

6

this difficulty and since then the research has proceeded fairly smoothly.

As far as we can see at this moment, the principal difficulty was caused by the realization that our old, well-proven methods had to be given up or, at any rate, considerably modified because of the new conditions. In order to highlight this important clash, we characterized the old method as that of the 'great detective' and the new that of 'tuning in' or experiencing a 'flash'.

The doctor using the technique of the great detective 'listened' most intently, observed everything carefully and, if necessary, examined conscientiously every area which, in his opinion, might be involved in the patient's problems. In a metaphorical sense this meant that he could 'leave no stone unturned'. Of course, this conscientious work needed considerable time, hence the technique of the 'long interviews'. The introduction of the focal therapy into general practice meant still more exacting standards for the 'great detective'. He was expected not only to 'listen' most carefully but also to use his observations so skilfully that he needed no longer to turn up every stone but infer unfailingly which stones had to be turned up to provide all the necessary clues. In our first attempts we thought that this process could be speeded up so that one could carry out the treatment in 'mini-long interviews' lasting at most fifteen to twenty minutes.

Perhaps it should be mentioned here that the role of the great detective is very near to the doctor's traditional role in illness-centred medicine; this is especially true for the diagnostic period. This similarity was almost certainly a strong contributory factor to the difficulties experienced by some members of the research team when they realized that their accustomed ways of functioning would have to be revised. These traditional functions assure the doctor of a safe feeling of superiority: it is he who knows more, to whom the patient turns with hope and trust, and who can prove by the success of his diagnostic skills that the trust in his superior knowledge and skills was justified. Looking at the diagnostic period from this angle, every turned up stone yielding a clue is a most rewarding and reassuring experience to both partners in the doctor/patient relationship.

In our new technique all these rewarding and reassuring

7

experiences had to be given up. Instead of solving exciting puzzles and problems, the doctor was now expected to 'tune in' so exactly to the patient's wavelength of communications that he would be able to respond to them fairly faultlessly. This state of 'being tuned in' must be kept up for the whole length of the interview so that the doctor and patient may be able to talk to each other without much danger of a misunderstanding. Another way of describing the same experience of two minds 'clicking in' with each other is to call it experiencing a flash. We found that this flash might happen either in the patient, or in the doctor or, which proved to have the best therapeutic prospect, simultaneously in both of them.

Yet another way of describing this technique would be to contrast it with the old method. In this latter the doctor had the privilege and the responsibility *to understand* 'what the patient tried to convey to him', *to recognize* all the omissions and distortions in it, using his knowledge to solve them unfailingly and with his skill to enable the patient to produce the right associations which would prove that his solutions were, on the whole, correct. This role is that of a leader, of a superior. In the new technique the therapist's role is to 'tune in', to follow the patient's lead, to allow the patient to use the therapist, even to make use of him. This is definitely a less glamorous, more modest role.

I am afraid that the many metaphors used here, with their rather poetical atmosphere, may create mistrust in the reader and confound instead of helping him. My difficulty is that I have to describe experiences in the therapeutic relationship which are perhaps unfamiliar to most analysts. So may I interrupt the discussion at this point and present one of our cases which has been followed up for two years. After this I shall resume the discussion which can then be based on concrete clinical material.

The case will start with one individual member but it will soon become evident that it is, in fact, about a whole family. The individual member, Miss Oldham, joined Dr Green's list in 1967 when her previous doctor died. She was then sixty-eight, single, a retired clerk. She was living in a self-contained flat in her brother's house. He was about one year younger and had married late, a woman of about his own age. There was another self-contained flat in the house which was occupied by Miss Beverley, also a single woman, in her late fifties, a very close friend of Miss Oldham's; they spent a great deal of time in each other's company. Unlike Miss Oldham, these three people had been on the doctor's list for many years. One more important detail: when Miss Oldham's mother became seriously ill, well up in her nineties, Miss Oldham insisted that she should be transferred to her flat where they nursed her most devotedly until she died. The mother was also the doctor's patient, so he knew Miss Oldham very well indeed. He knew, for instance, that Miss Oldham was a kind woman, interested in church work, in helping people in trouble, but found cruelty and violence distasteful and revolting.

When joining the practice Miss Oldham came with a host of complaints which the doctor had some difficulty in sorting out. Eventually they could be traced back to a chronic overdose of Diamox, a potent drug prescribed for glaucoma by a consultant. When this drug was stopped all the symptoms disappeared. The doctor soon discovered also that the patient had been treated previously by two more consultants, so that he came to the conclusion that Miss Oldham was very likely somewhat over-anxious about her health. Then followed a completely uneventful period, Miss Oldham seeing the doctor at intervals of six to eight weeks.

In comparison, the medical records of the other members of the family are very slight. Mr Oldham, like his sister, is good-looking, well-preserved, and always well-dressed. He has had only minor illnesses like bronchitis; in fact, he is hardly ever ill. In contrast to him, his wife looks much older and has some anginal pains. The last member of this set-up, Miss Beverley, is a somewhat tense and anxious woman but, apart from occasional colds, she has usually been well. Of course, she knows all the members of the Oldham family intimately.

In the summer of 1968 Miss Oldham appeared again, complaining of being under the weather, of poor sleep and some giddiness. After a thorough physical examination the doctor came to the traditional diagnosis of anxiety and depression.

Although Dr Green had known that she—like her mother—ever since her childhood had suffered, especially during weekends, from migrainous headaches which considerably interfered with her enjoyment of life, until this interview he did not try to probe

9

deeper into Miss Oldham's possible personal problems. Thinking that this was an opportune moment, he asked her what she could tell him about herself. First she said, 'Nothing,' but then slowly it could be established that Miss Oldham had often been ill in the past; that she was afraid of violence and of becoming a burden to other people, that she and Miss Beverley were very close friends, that she used to be equally friendly with her brother, but when she brought her mother to the house her brother became jealous of the intimacy between the two women. At this point the doctor probed further, asking whether the brother's marriage had made any difference to her, to which she gave an evasive answer. Instead of pressing further, Dr Green felt that he had gone too far and said 'All right, let's leave it there'. The atmosphere changed and they both seemed aware of it. The doctor stopped here because he thought that the patient had told him as much as she could and at this moment any attempt to get more from her would cause serious resistances. He felt that during this interview he and his patient got on to a 'different level' and this was acknowledged by both of them, though without any words.

May I repeat here that every case reported became a research case and was followed up systematically at periods of ten to eighteen months. Right from the start we accepted the principle that without explicit predictions in the initial phase no follow-up could verify or refute any idea. With this principle in mind, each doctor was asked to state in his initial report which was recorded and then transcribed: (1) two diagnoses for each case—the traditional and the overall diagnosis, (2) his therapeutic plans for both, and (3) his predictions for both.

In Miss Oldham's case the traditional diagnosis was: migraine, general tension, insomnia. The overall diagnosis was: (1) very strong family ties, obligation to care for other people; (2) fear of cruelty and violence; (3) secretiveness about her own emotional and sexual life, possibly only weak heterosexual urges with some —more or less conscious—homosexual ones; (4) tension between brother and sister, possibly because of jealousy: (a) about mother (b) about sister-in-law (c) about Miss Beverley.

The doctor added that, realizing that Miss Oldham expected to receive some medication for her presenting symptoms—the tradi-

10

tional diagnosis—he prescribed some hypnotic and some tonic, while the treatment for the overall diagnosis consisted of showing to the patient: (a) that there was no need between them to use pretence organic illnesses if she wanted some help from him, and (b) that he had some idea of what sort of problems the patient was struggling with but he was in no hurry to force her to talk about them right now. For the future his plan was to explore with his patient how far she could—and needed to—talk about her intimate problems.

The first response by Miss Oldham was very encouraging. She made an appointment to see Dr Green a week later when she started, perhaps to test the doctor's sincerity, by complaining in the old way about another attack of migraine. As the doctor just waited, she changed her approach and added that her attacks of migraine spoilt her enjoyment of life, and then started to talk about her fear of becoming a burden, no matter to whom; she must feel that she had done her duty and not given offence. Then she said, 'I've been thinking a lot about what you said about my secretiveness,' and added that, in fact, she had not talked much about herself until now. A pause followed, tolerated by both of them, and then quite unexpectedly she said, 'You remind me of my father'.

Then came a long story about her mild father and her stern mother who used to be cross with him and tell him off, whereupon Father left the room but used to creep back, asking meekly, 'Are you still cross with me?' The doctor admitted that at first he was not very pleased to be felt so meek and mild but then he realized that there was no criticism, only affection, in Miss Oldham's story. She talked about her brothers who were similar to their mother and saw to it that she had her corners knocked off. Dr Green commented here that perhaps these experiences were the reason why she got on so much better with women than with men; she thought a bit and then agreed that this might be so. After a while the doctor asked what sort of tension was in the house, was it true that Miss Oldham was jealous of her sister-in-law, and he learned that, quite to the contrary, the sister-in-law was jealous of the close friendship between the two spinsters, Miss Oldham and Miss Beverley.

On questioning, he reported that on this occasion he did not find it necessary to prescribe anything, although the patient started the

11

session by complaining about her migraines. Apparently the patient did not expect anything either since she went away quite satisfied.

The doctor was able to state his predictions more explicitly. These were: (1) it is very likely that Miss Oldham will maintain the 'new level' in her relationship with the doctor provided (2) the doctor does not try to push and hurry her; (3) probably she will continue to offer all sorts of somatic 'illnesses' (4) but these will not be very impressive provided the doctor will take them seriously but not allow her to get off the 'new level', that is, back to her absolute secretiveness.

As already stated, it is an integral part of our research to follow up systematically at regular intervals all the patients who have been reported to our seminars. Miss Oldham's turn came about 11 months after she had first been reported. During this period Miss Oldham was seen only four times—as I have just mentioned, she used to see the doctor every 6–8 weeks. During the same time her friend, Miss Beverley, was seen twice—about the average— and her brother four times, definitely more than average, while her sister-in-law was not seen at all.

There was an undramatic though steady development in Miss Oldham's relationship with her doctor. Each time she presented some apparently organic complaints and each time she seemed to welcome it that no organic cause could be found. The 'different level' was maintained, she talked more freely about herself, but it was always she who decided when to stop. First she admitted that since the discussions she could be more self-assertive, especially with her brother. At a later visit she mentioned that she used to be dominated by her brother who thought he was always right, although usually he was not; now she had no difficulty in remaining firm with him. Although she still hated and disliked violence, this was somewhat better now, but her fear of becoming ill and a burden to other people was still very strong. However, all this was said in a way that the doctor could not make use of. Still, he tried to enquire about the influence of possible stresses at home but she brushed it off, saying that now she could be much more forceful than before and now there were no stresses.

Remarkably, Miss Beverley, out of the blue, told the doctor her whole life history. It was obvious that the two women must have discussed what had happened between Miss Oldham and Dr Green. Very likely, Miss Beverley wanted to have equal treatment but only if she could be sure that the doctor would leave her alone. Apart from this, she confirmed that Miss Oldham could now stand up for herself.

The brother's visits were for only minor illnesses, like singing in the ears, slight bronchitis etc. Each time he mentioned that his sister was much more lively in everything she did and that it was much to his liking.

In the next follow-up period Miss Oldham's case was brought up for discussion fifteen months after the first follow-up report. During this time Mr and Mrs Oldham did not consult Dr Green at all, Miss Oldham saw him five times and so did Miss Beverley.

The frequency of Miss Oldham's attendances remained the same as in the previous follow-up period, i.e. one in every three months. She came complaining of sleeplessness, influenza, and in the post-influenzal period of some gastritis. There was no complaint of migraine, of being run down, or any other signs of depression. Dr Green felt that the tension had been considerably reduced and apparently reverted to his old ways because he gave her some hypnotics for her sleeplessness and a mixture of magnesia for her gastritis. It will be remembered that in his therapeutic plan given two years ago he decided not to give drugs if this could be avoided.

Apparently the relationship between brother and sister had settled on a new level because he was not mentioned at all. Instead of him, Miss Beverley was mentioned several times as being bossy and difficult, especially just before the holiday which all of them were taking together. When returning from holiday, things in this relationship seem to have become calmer, because Miss Oldham reported that although Miss Beverley was difficult she could tolerate it. Miss Beverley came five times during this period which was definitely more frequent than her average. She complained of an irritating itching in her skin and some other annoying minor symptoms. She was anxious that the doctor should appreciate that life for her was hard and she had to suffer. This he did and then tried to use the opportunity to let her talk of her life history which she presented to him out of the blue about a year ago, but she responded evasively.

One more important detail must be mentioned here. After the clearing up of the symptoms of the Diamox overdose during which there was fairly close collaboration between Dr Green and the ophthalmic surgeon, the two doctors had no contact with each other. Dr Green assumed that Miss Oldham, as all his glaucoma patients, went on having periodic checks with the surgeon, but did not bother to find out more about it. About February 1970 he received a note from the surgeon informing him that as the intraocular tension in Miss Oldham's eye had become somewhat high and could not be reduced by medication, an iris inclusion would be performed in a couple of weeks. The operation was successful, the tension was reduced and her sight got a bit better.

What happened in this case? An intimidated and frightened spinster who had never been able to express her real feelings was enabled to get in touch with herself, to become aware of some of her feelings of guilt and shame, and to talk about them up to a point. The principal topics that she was helped with were: her love for her meek father, her dislike of her domineering mother and brothers; her dislike of violent scenes on the one hand and her fear of becoming weak and dependent on the other; and lastly her dislike of being alone. These were all secrets which almost certainly had never been mentioned to anyone. The patient's reponse to this ventilation was (a) less frequent visits to the doctor, (b) less insistence on presenting organic illnesses, and (c) a definite change in her subdued behaviour towards a more realistic self-assertiveness. As she brushed aside a number of tentative overtures by the doctor, he decided to accept for the time being what had been achieved and not to press for more.

During a period of two years the results as described in the previous paragraph were maintained. Miss Oldham used the doctor at the reduced rate of about once in three months, she was able to make peace with her brother without giving up her newly gained self-assertiveness; she became able to talk about the strains in her relationship to Miss Beverley and perhaps through this she could tolerate these strains better. Her lifelong attacks of migraine have completely gone for the time being as well as the feeling of being run down and all other symptoms of a mild depression.

14

Everything points to a considerable reduction of tension in Miss Oldham's condition except one single detail which is the increase of intraocular tension in her glaucomatous eye, necessitating an operation. Glaucoma is definitely a candidate for a place among the psychosomatic illnesses although the evidence is not yet convincing. If this proposition is rejected, we need not bother more: in a case of chronic simple glaucoma one iris inclusion at seventy, especially if Diamox cannot be used, is a fairly normal event. If, on the other hand, we accept the idea of a psychosomatic condition, the possibility of the tension being removed from all other spheres of life and being accumulated in the eyes cannot be excluded altogether. We know that Dr Green did not bother to keep up a close contact with the surgeon and did not do anything even after he received the information about the coming operation. It must be added that this would be a fairly normal procedure between a general practitioner and one of his consultants who had got to know and trust each other. Still we have to ask, as was done in the seminar, would it have made a difference if Dr Green had watched the changes in the intraocular tension together with the surgeon? We do not know the answer but the case will be followed up.

In spite of this uncertain detail, this is definitely an acceptable result, considering that she is a seventy-year-old spinster who has never had any contact with a man and has retired from work for some years. This result was achieved in two sessions, each lasting ten to fifteen minutes, say in thirty minutes: even if we add to this figure the nine follow-up or continuation sessions, we reach the sum total of eleven sessions of ten to fifteen minutes' duration. amounting to a total time given to the patient of less than three hours. I ought to add that we have about forty cases of this kind, recorded and followed-up in the same way as Miss Oldham's. This means that these results are not due to chance but can be aimed at and achieved with a fair amount of certainty. On the other hand this does not mean that this sort of therapy can be done with all our cases and at all times; it must be remembered that our cases are not a representative sample because the doctors were requested to report only patients with whom they thought they had been able to achieve something; it is readily admitted that even among this selected sample we had a fair proportion of failures. Still, by now, we can say that our techniques work in a number of cases.

The technique used by Dr Green is a fair illustration of what we call flash technique or that of accepting the patient's lead, of being used by the patient. There was not much 'detective' work in Miss Oldham's case: the few questions that Dr Green asked yielded hardly any useful material. This is especially true of his repeated enquiry about Miss Oldham's possible jealousy of her sister-in-law —a good illustration of our principle: he who asks questions gets answers but hardly anything else. Very few interpretations were made, perhaps the only important one being his startling remark about Miss Oldham not having told him much about herself.

As far as one can see, the therapeutic work was done chiefly by 'tuning in' to the patient, understanding her communications and responding to them so that she would feel that she was understood. Of course, a good deal of this happened by verbal communication between the two, but in this reciprocal communication and under-standing the dictionary meanings of the words played only a minor role; one could say that understanding of what Miss Oldham did not say in words was about as important as the understanding of what she actually said. It has to be added that the same was true about the doctor's communications. In spite of all this, the 'different level' could be established and maintained, at any rate in the two years of the follow-up, without either of the two partners having even mentioned it in so many words.

Parallel with this verbal/non-verbal way of communicating there happened very little examination of the patient's psychopathology. One knows that the two spinsters were very close friends but that is about all; ideas like mother-fixation, homosexuality, either overt or covert, etc., were not touched upon nor even hinted at; equally, the relationship between her fear of violence and her possible passionateness or the intensity of her instinctual drive etc., was not even enquired into. In spite of this lack of proper data, real therapy could be decided upon and carried out.

Admittedly this lack of proper foundation for planning the therapy and then carrying it out had certain undeniable dangers. The first group of dangers is caused by the high degree of identi-fication with the patient which is demanded from the doctor by our new technique. Evidently the very fine 'tuning in', leading to a flash, can be achieved only if the doctor is capable of a very far-reaching identification with the patient. We analysts have learnt how much this sort of identification can help in the therapy of a difficult case, but also that it may lead, especially with certain patients, to most hazardous developments in the doctor/patient relationship. Being controlled by the patient, unconscious and therefore uncontrolled collusion, leading to a relationship reminiscent of a veritable *folie à deux*, are only a few of these undesirable and dangerous developments. I think it should be mentioned here that some of these and related developments have been extensively studied by the Kleinians under the heading of 'projective identification'.

It is generally agreed that the best prevention against these dangers is a successfully terminated personal analysis for the therapist. Since none of the doctors taking part in this research has had this, their accident proneness in this direction must be rated high. This danger expressed as being taken possession of or being used by a patient, is a constant preoccupation in the minds of most general practitioners and therefore it is likely that we erred by being over-cautious. As Miss Oldham's case shows, Dr Green accepted his patient's lead very well indeed but only up to a point; the identification with Miss Oldham was excellent during the first period of the follow-up but became less intense and less reliable in the second. Possibly this reverting to prescribing drugs in the second period must be considered as a symptom of his less reliable identification. The same cautious attitude was evident in several others of our cases reported by other doctors.

This leads me to an important problem of our research which we are beginning to study at present: what is the right continuation of a really successful flash? Should the doctor rely on further flashes occurring in the subsequent interviews or will it be sufficient for him to continue in the later interviews by reverting to the role of the 'detective' or to some sort of focal technique—especially if he does not experience a further flash? Alternatively, if no flash occurs in a subsequent interview, should he take it as a sign that at the moment he should be patient and should not try to do anything important? All these, and many more alternatives, are being

17

studied at this moment and as we do not have the answers as yet I must plead for patience.

Now let us turn to the discussion of what we psychoanalysts can learn from these observations and experiences. Let us start with what we already know, which is that transference is ubiquitous. Miss Oldham told the doctor that he reminded her of her father; to which we can add that Dr Green is still this side of his fiftieth year while Miss Oldham is nearly seventy. This of course was not an intellectual recognition of some similarity but a communication highly charged with emotion—a true transference manifestation. What perhaps will interest us most is that Dr Green, after some conscious hesitation, was able to handle this transference situation; he understood it and used its therapeutic possibilities in a skilful way—without wasting one word on it. This proves that even non-analysed people, if properly trained, can learn to understand not too complex transference manifestations and make use of them for therapy. A further important detail is that all this could be done without any difficulty in spite of the fact that the doctor had just examined Miss Oldham's body. I have discussed on several occasions how some of our well-tested findings obtained in the psychoanalytical situation must be re-examined for any new setting.

The remark I wish to make is about the similarity between Winnicott's diagnostic therapeutic interviews and our techniques. Of course the two analyst leaders have known Winnicott's approach for a long time—in fact we invited him to talk about it to the Focal Therapy Workshop in the mid-fifties—and have followed its development ever since. Although influenced by his ideas, we started out on our research unprepared for our experiences leading our work in this direction. The similarity is still more surprising if one considered that Winnicott's approach presupposes a highly trained and most sensitive psychoanalyst-paediatrician, while our colleagues are general practitioners with no particular analytic training. Nevertheless the similarity is there.

CHAPTER 2

The 'Flash' Technique —
Its Freedom and Its Discipline[1]

ENID BALINT

This chapter will describe some aspects of the flash technique with special reference to the discipline and the freedom which they give to the doctor.

Three working principles have emerged from this kind of work. The first working principle is that the doctor should not be too preoccupied either with theories or preconceived questions arising from these theories (however vague and unobtrusive they may seem to him) because if he is he may either fail to notice obvious and simple events in the interview, or if he notices them will not spontaneously remember them; he may be reminded of them by the discussion in the seminar but otherwise they may remain unavailable for therapy or he will judge them as too unimportant to use.

For all these reasons the therapeutic work may concentrate on relatively unimportant aspects or side-issues of the patient's problems.

The usual questions in a doctor's mind when he is doing traditional illness-centred medicine (be it physical or psychological) are 'Where is the illness located?' and 'What caused it?' In psychotherapy the causation of illness is usually looked for in the relationship with parents and siblings, i.e. in early childhood. In the flash technique these questions and the observations which might help to answer them do not have a privileged position. But, as we know,

[1] A shortened version of this paper was read in Paris at the International Congress of the Société Française de Médicine Psychosomatique in September 1970 and published in the *Revue de Médicine Psychosomatique et de Psychologie Médicale*, No. 3, 1970.

19

it is very difficult to observe anything in an interview when there is no available theory to explain it, no half ready jig-saw puzzle into which to insert a neat piece when what is observed apparently makes no sense. If one has a theory, one is limited by the theory; if one has no theory, it is difficult to observe . . . but it gives freedom to observe. This freedom is useful only if it is coupled with discipline: in our case the discipline of careful and attentive observations, and the ability to know how much of what is observed originated with the patient and how much is contributed by the doctor himself.

The second working principle concerns what the doctor would do with his observations. This, oddly enough, is less difficult. The difficulty is more in keeping up the intensity of attentive observation after a decision has been made to comment or interpret. In other ways (and perhaps in this way too) our technique is similar to all others in psychotherapy. The doctor has to reflect silently about his observations and their meaning: identify with the patient, develop ideas about him, and then intervene by making a comment or interpretation to test out his line of thought. As we know, the observing, silent reflecting part of the process is done very rapidly. There is, however, no hurry for comment. In fact the comment can only be useful if the doctor and patient are both working, both concentrating on a common task. The patient may respond to any comment suggested by the doctor even if it turns out at a later date not to be central to his problems at that particular time. There is in fact always the danger that the patient will be only too pleased to respond to the doctor's ideas and get away from his own 'irrational' ones. In the kind of work we are describing it is more important to make contact with what is bothering the patient at the moment at which the interview is taking place, even if it seems peripheral to his main problem, than to tackle what might be more basic disturbances. This kind of work sometimes leads to silences but we have found that even the ten to fifteen minutes available to the doctor during office hours is enough to allow for silences which only seem long if the intensity of the attention between the doctor and the patient is great.

The third working principle concerns the doctor's respect for the patient's right to hide—not to disclose his secrets: in fact, respect for the patient's privacy. Our technique does not involve trying to break through defences. If the doctor observes that the patient is hiding some feeling—or half showing, half hiding—is ill at ease, over assertive, hesitant etc. etc.— his primary aim is *not* to get in touch with the secret, but to test whether his assumptions are correct. The doctor must give the patient the *opportunity* to communicate. If the offer is accepted and a flash occurs in the patient which is responded to by the doctor, the doctor is in duty bound to discipline himself to continue to observe the patient's and his own contributions to the therapeutic process—but not to run after secrets, which blunts his ability to observe what is there before his eyes. You may ask what is the use of all this. If the aim of therapy is not to find out what caused the illness, what is it for? Will this kind of technique help the patient?

Our experience shows that if these working principles are more or less adhered to, an intense, intimate contact is sometimes made between the doctor and the patient. This contact does not lead to a dependent clinging relationship, or to a strong transference neurosis. But the flash of understanding, if meaningful, may expose the tip of an iceberg, or the heat of a fiery cauldron, which, perhaps, over the weeks or months or years can gradually be explored either by the patient and doctor together or by the patient alone, and the patient then finds he can make more use of himself and of his environment. The patient's independence and human dignity are not endangered. He feels (and is) in control of the situation. He can use the doctor when he wishes within the limits that the doctor's personality, technique and skill allow. The patient is in control of the pace and content of the therapy. The patient (and sometimes the doctor too) may make links between present problems and early childhood difficulties, but we think in this technique the links consolidate the work but are not in themselves the therapeutic tool. The therapy, we think, lies in the peculiar intense flash of understanding between the doctor and patient in a setting where an ongoing contact is possible, where neither the doctor nor the patient gives up his self-esteem. The patient's ego functioning is enhanced, rather than diminished. One could say he becomes more 'full of himself', accepting, though not necessarily condoning, his failures, weaknesses and strengths.

I will now describe a fragment of a case which I reported in some detail in a previous paper.[2] At the time of the initial report by the doctor in June 1967 our thinking did not permit us to discuss the work in the terms I have been using. It was before we discovered the importance of the flash but, as I shall show, the word was used during the discussion of the follow-up of the case three years later in June 1970.

A patient of Dr Black's, Mrs Salford, was fifty-six in 1967. Her most frequent complaint over the fifteen years the doctor had known her had been tension headaches. When the doctor reported the case he said he wished to do so because 'though he had known the patient for fifteen years she had never become alive to him before this interview'. He said 'this patient had been a type before and had now become a person in this interview'. The seminar said that this should really be our criterion for our ten-minute psychotherapy, which was how at the beginning of this research we described the psychotherapy which was done in ordinary office hours. In his overall diagnosis the doctor said that Mrs Salford was an unhappy, frustrated woman. His therapeutic decision was to bring some of her feelings out into the open—'to see why she had to drive herself to breaking point all the time'. We soon realized that this was the kind of patient who would be driven away by questions and that she was not anyway the kind of case most doctors would want to take on for long interviews.

The next phase of therapy which started three months later consisted of three very dynamic interviews lasting respectively ten minutes, twenty minutes and ten minutes over a period of three weeks. During this phase the patient was enabled to discover that her husband loved her and this allowed her to work less hard and her headaches disappeared. We predicted that the patient would be able to continue to communicate with her husband. After this episode the patient only visited the doctor four times before the next follow-up discussion in the seminar, which was in May 1969. The doctor then said we had been right and that communication had been kept up between the husband and the wife and that the

[2] 'The Possibilities of Patient-centred Medicine', Journal of Royal College of General Practitioners, 1969, Vol. 17.

patient looked more feminine and still showed that she knew that her husband loved her. Balint at this time said that he thought that this was exactly what our research started with, that is to say it demonstrated what we wanted to study; 'the doctor felt that something had really happened at the first interview. . . . We had used all sorts of similes: a light had been switched on; a curtain was raised; something *happened*—not that the doctor did something but that something happened.' It was however a year later, in June 1970 at the next follow-up discussion, that Balint said 'this is the first case that might be called a flash.'

To return to the May 1969 follow-up discussions. At the time the patient came to the doctor following a road accident in which she had been hurt by a motor cyclist when crossing the road. Her leg had been injured and she had been taken to hospital. There was no bone injury. She made little of the incident and laughingly said that she was more concerned about the motor cyclist (who was unhurt) than about herself. The doctor noticed the mockery and insincerity but said nothing. The patient then went on to tell him what happened at the casualty department at the hospital where she was taken after the accident. The doctor told us that the patient was so funny when recounting this episode that he couldn't help laughing. She had been disoriented but no-one had comforted her or helped her. This communication led the doctor to stop the funny story (which could have been taken to mean that she could cope very well and needed no help) but he did not try to take the work further. The patient then said. 'Funny thing I haven't had a single headache for ages. I wonder why. . . .'

The following question was then asked. Should the doctor have taken the opportunity given him when she said she had had no headaches for ages and linked this change with his earlier interviews? This question, I think, highlights the fact that there are usually many points in an interview which are ignored and which, if taken up, might lead to a flash. Some go unnoticed—some are noticed and ignored by every doctor. Would for instance the intensity of a flash have occurred if our doctor had made a comment following the funny story before the patient spoke about the headaches? He felt he should have done so. He said however, 'I was pleased to let well alone.' This feeling in the doctor (let's

23

leave well alone; something good has happened, I had better be careful not to spoil it) frequently occurs in our kind of work. We do not yet know if it is not an essential feature of the flash technique (that is to say a very cautious, non-interfering attitude) or whether it should be overcome, when even better results will be achieved. The doctor himself said that the case was one where he first became aware of the difficulty of the follow-up in a flash case. He said he got into a rut and did not know what to do. The importance of the research into what to do with a successful flash case or after a successful flash interview was emphasised. Is the doctor under an obligation to continue at the next encounter? Is he wrong and failing in his duty if he does not, or is it an unwarranted intrusion into the patient's life if the doctor tries to elicit a flash on the next occasion? We do not know the answer to these questions, but we do feel that we must not exploit former successes or intrude unnecessarily. However, perhaps I should come back to my opening remarks, namely that the doctor must not be too preoccupied with theories or preconceived questions arising from these theories—even if these arise out of theories about the flash technique—so that he may fail to notice simple and obvious events which are going on in the present.

What is special about this technique? Many may feel that the only difference between our flash technique and any 'normal' psychotherapy is in our setting in which interviews must be brief. I do not know whether this is true, as we do not yet know for certain whether the intensity of the brief general practitioner interviews can be transplanted to different settings where longer interviews are normal, but where an ongoing contact over the years is not.

To *summarize*, I think the main characteristics of our technique are:

1. In the intensity of the contact;
2. In the freedom it gives to the patient to use the doctor in his own way;
3. In the freedom it gives to the doctor to make his own observations;
4. In the freedom it gives to the doctor to be used, i.e. to give himself, without anxiety that his patients will abuse his time;

5. In the discipline it imposes on the doctor during the brief interviews to observe both the patient and his own thoughts and feelings.

In our work the doctor is freed from the primary task of trying to discover *why* the patient talks, thinks, feels and behaves in the way he does. The patient in due course may provide the answers to *why*; the doctor's task is primarily to observe a very small sample of *how* the patient talks, thinks and behaves, and *why* this causes him pain; *what* he is like and what he seeks in an obscure and confused way to share with his doctor; what really makes him want the doctor's attention. May I add that this aspect of our work has nothing to do with solving problems or averting crises. And it is a very hard and disciplined work indeed.

This method can perhaps be taught best by the way the seminar leaders behave by creating an atmosphere where such freedom and discipline exists; where it is not the leader who knows the answers, but where his observations are as free and his attention as complete and his thinking as disciplined as that required by the doctors in their interviews with their patients. This is again a very difficult task indeed.

CHAPTER 3

The Patient's Use of His Doctor[1]

H. STEPHEN PASMORE

In January 1966, Enid and Michael Balint invited a group of general practitioners, who had participated for many years in their seminars, to join a research team. The aim of the research was to find out new techniques to enable general practitioners to offer psychological help to their patients during the course of a ten-minute interview, without adversely affecting the normal routine of their practices.

In order to categorize the findings of the research team and to enable suitable comparisons between cases to be made, two forms were drawn up—one for the initial report on the case, and another for the follow-up. One of the most important items on each form was concerned with the Overall Diagnosis—a diagnosis based on the psychological as well as the physical aspects of the case being reported. For example, a typical overall diagnosis that was given in a seminar in the case of a widow, who had left and obtained a divorce from her first husband and whose second husband had died, and who was now complaining of depression was 'An unfeminine, insecure but apparently competent widow. Her efficiency may have caused her loneliness as well as being an escape for her from it. She probably felt guilty over what had happened to the husbands, whom she probably crushed, and guilty that she had treated her daughters overbearingly as her mother had treated her. Now

[1] This chapter was read as a paper at the First International Conference of the Balint Society in March, 1972.

the daughters were growing up she could not always escape from being lonely.'

Now the members of the seminar become very proficient at making such an overall diagnosis, but at this time they were only able to do so by asking their patients many questions. This approach to the patient was fostered by the rivalry of the members who demanded every scrap of information possible from the doctor presenting the case in order to come to an opinion about it. This led later to the coining of the phrase 'detective inspector' to describe the doctor whose technique was to range over the whole of the patient's life to enable a good overall diagnosis to be made.

In March 1968, after the the seminar had been in progress for $2\frac{1}{4}$ years, Balint drew the doctors' attention to the fact that virtually no progress had been made on the research project itself. The doctors, on the other hand, felt they had made a lot of progress with their own skills though they had not fully come to terms with their disappointment at failing to make close contact with their patients through those newly acquired skills.

In this connection it is interesting to recall that Balint had described how difficult it was for the doctors attending his seminars for the first time to abandon their apostolic function of thinking they knew best how their patients should behave once they had been consulted by them for advice, 'and what was right and what was wrong for patients to expect and endure.' In 1968 the doctors in the seminar did not see that in becoming proficient in making an overall diagnosis they had acquired a second apostolic function related to their psychological skills, which had replaced their first apostolic function related to their medical skills in treating organic diseases.

After this intervention by Balint, which was very dramatic when it occurred, the members of the seminar began to work in a different way. They found they could abandon the second apostolic function they had acquired and instead become more sensitive to their patients' needs and more attentive to what their patient was trying to say. They were able to 'tune-in' more often to the same wavelength as their patient, so that there was no longer any necessity to probe like a detective into all the patient's affairs. They began to practise 'selective attention and selective neglect'

27

D

which Balint had tried out in his focal therapy workshop some years previously. They moved from thinking in terms of one-person psychology to two-person psychology; in other words, they were able to get closer to the patient by exploring the doctor/patient relationship rather than the patient's psychopathology. They began to see the patient in a new light and try to help him from a new angle. Instead of thinking how they could best examine, diagnose and treat their patients, the doctors began to ask themselves how their patients could best use them.

The patient's use of the doctor can well be studied in the following case, which was reported by Dr Sage in October 1969 at the time when the seminar was beginning to move away from the detective-inspector position.

Mrs Thornbury was a housewife aged thirty-one, married for fourteen years to a milk roundsman aged thirty-eight and who had six children aged from four to thirteen. She had been on the doctor's list for three-and-a-half years, and was the eldest daughter of a family of six, all well known to the doctor's practice. Mrs Thornbury's father had died of cancer of the bronchus two years previously. Her mother was sluttish but pleasant, and managed to get her daughter and family put on the doctor's list in spite of the fact that they were outside the doctor's usual practice area.

Mrs Thornbury was an anxious woman who was concerned about her children, but who gave a superficial air of coping well. In February 1968 she had to spend three days in hospital for an acute anxiety state, which the doctor later found was associated with her getting pregnant for the seventh time, and a little later she was admitted to hospital for termination of the pregnancy, and sterilization at her request. She was under the hospital psychiatrists for a few weeks, both before and after the termination. She consulted the doctor early the next year, wondering why her psoriasis was spreading, but gave nothing away about her real anxieties. The doctor noted her husband was thinking of buying a larger council house, where her mother, who had some hypertension, might be able to live with them. At the same time, Mrs Thornbury confided to the doctor that she had thought of fostering babies now she could not have any more, but half smiled when she added that no-one would allow it.

The Patient's Use of His Doctor

In the ten minute interview reported to the seminar Mrs Thornbury started by saying that she felt tired and irritable. 'I'm so tired and I wake up in the middle of the night and I'm fed up'. The doctor immediately thought she was worried that she could not have any more babies, but Mrs Thornbury went on to say that she was concerned as her husband also woke in the middle of the night, and this was upsetting as he had to get up between five and six a.m. to go to work. The doctor asked what the husband did when he awoke, and Mrs Thornbury replied that he said he was sorry that she was awake, and turned over to go to sleep again. 'Couldn't he have made love to you?' asked the doctor, determined to ferret out the facts. 'Oh no,' Mrs Thornbury replied, 'nothing like that; I'm not so keen on that. You know I'm really frigid' and she gave a raucous laugh. 'Frigid, with all those children?' said the doctor. 'Well yes, I've never liked sex. I've only endured it because I knew I would be able to have a baby afterwards'. At this stage Mrs Thornbury seems to have engaged the doctor, for he found himself looking at her and noticing how attractively dressed she was. He remarked on it, and she laughed and said she got a lot of wolf whistles when she walked down the road. 'But don't you ever have sex with your husband?' the doctor persisted. 'You've got to be careful as the children might hear,' she replied, avoiding a straight answer.

In his overall diagnosis the doctor described Mrs Thornbury as an immature person who enjoyed babies rather than children, and played with them as if they were dolls. She had married young and had never reached the stage of truly adult functioning as her husband mothered her too. She had never got over the death of her father.

In summarizing the interview, the doctor felt it had been frigid, with the patient tightening up in response to his pushing too hard.

Mrs Thornbury made an emergency appointment to see the doctor a week later as her son aged seven had been sent home from school that day with severe abdominal pain. The doctor examined the boy and found nothing abnormal physically, and then looked at his notes to find that the boy had had a similar pain about twenty-five times previously and had been investigated at two hospitals when younger. The doctor asked Mrs Thornbury

29

what she thought had provoked the pain this time, and she said her son had come home very late from school the previous evening and she had been very worried that he might have been knocked down and killed. She was very angry with him and as he was always upset when she was angry with him she thought that might have precipitated his pain. The doctor found Mrs Thornbury looking at him with what he could only describe as 'a teasing smile of triumph'. He was a little annoyed; 'So you really knew what it was, didn't you?' he said. 'Yes I did, but I wanted to be absolutely sure,' she replied.

This case shows how difficult it is for the doctor to make close contact with his patient when using the technique of the detective-inspector; for while this technique enables the doctor to make a good overall diagnosis, it does not help him to find out what the patient really needs at the moment the patient seeks his help. In studying the case, it is plain to see how the doctor used the patient but not how the patient used the doctor. The doctor used the patient to find out her probable anxieties connected with her inability to have further babies as a result of her sterilization. The doctor's questions were directed to that end as he thought this would be the most useful focus on which he could work with the patient. The patient, on the other hand, was using the doctor in a different way. She appeared to be trying to bolster up her defences against her anxieties, whatever they stemmed from, rather than showing any desire to work with the doctor to gain a better understanding of herself.

In making a closer study of the case it can be seen that Mrs Thornbury started by making a direct statement to the doctor about her state of mind. She felt 'tired and irritable'. She went on to relate her tiredness to waking up in the middle of the night and saying she was fed-up with it. On the surface this appeared to be a direct communication about the state of her sexual relations with her husband; and the doctor, knowing of her love of babies and of her recent sterilization, jumped to the conclusion that she was worried that she could not have any more babies. But Mrs Thornbury went on to say that she was concerned that her wakefulness made her husband wake up. Did this in fact represent a fear that her husband would want intercourse with her if she were awake?

When asked how her husband reacted if she woke him, she replied that her husband said he was sorry she was awake and turned over to try to get asleep again. The doctor tried to probe deeper and suggested that her husband must occasionally make love to her, but she shrugged off his remarks with a raucous laugh, saying she was frigid and only endured sex in the hope of becoming pregnant. There had been quarrels with her husband because she did not want to have intercourse with him. Is it possible that one of her needs to have babies was to get pregnant so that she would have a good excuse not to have intercourse with her husband?

At this stage in the interview Mrs Thornbury was looking so attractive that she provoked the doctor to comment on her looks. 'But don't you ever have sex with your husband?' he said, which was the same as saying 'But can't a man enjoy sex with an attractive woman like you?' 'No, the children might hear,' she replied, or, in other words, 'It's forbidden' or 'I'm not going to let you near me.'

The patient's pattern of defences suggested she was worried about her frigidity and of being seen as an unfeminine sort of person. She made herself attractive to men, but kept them at a distance because of her uncertainty about herself as a woman and her fear of being rejected and getting hurt. She hated close contact with men for that threatened to expose her feeling of frigidity.

It is significant that Mrs Thornbury made an urgent appointment a week later to ask the doctor to examine her son for an acute abdominal pain, though she herself knew that her son had had similar attacks and that she was the cause of them. Was Mrs Thornbury trying to say to the doctor that as she thought he had seen through her bluff about her frigidity he might as well see how she provoked stress symptoms in her son and get some relief from confessing it? Or was she making herself attractive to the doctor by flattering him about his skill at carrying out a physical examination, and after he had carried out the examination making him look a fool by saying she knew that her son's symptoms were psychological all the time? Certainly, the doctor felt the latter interpretation was the correct one and that this was the constant pattern of her behaviour with men.

To sum up, it is clear that in the above case both doctor and

31

patient were on two completely different wavelengths. The doctor responded to the patient's complaint of tiredness and irritability by carrying out a skilful psychological examination using the detective-inspector technique, but though the doctor gained much interesting information about the patient and was able to make a good overall diagnosis, and no doubt gave the patient considerable help, he was unable to engage her closely or explore the nature of her underlying anxieties. He seemed to be offering the patient more than she herself wanted at the time.

The results of trying to help the patient by making a better overall diagnosis were not therefore found entirely satisfactory by the seminar, and it was found necessary to make a different approach to the patient. The seminar shifted their emphasis from the study of how the doctor could best help the patient to a study of how the patient could best use the doctor. The doctors found they had to keep themselves more in the background and yet listen more intently to what their patients were trying to say. They had to identify themselves more often with their patients and experience their deep feelings. They had to become more aware of the doctor/patient relationship and interpret the patient's past and present in terms of that relationship. They had to practice selective attention and selective neglect. In other words, to give of their best the doctors found they had to behave towards their patients in much the same way as Michael Balint behaved towards the members of his seminars.

CHAPTER 4

Types of Interview in General Practice: 'The Flash'

CYRIL GILL

The doctors in this research group were already experienced in long interviews on selected patients in their practices, whom they tried to help with personal problems. Our aim in the present research was to examine the ordinary 10-minute GP interview and see what we were able to do in such short contacts. There are many possible types of interaction between GP and patient. One might distinguish the following three categories with an example of each.

1. *Traditional medical interview*

A fifty-six-year-old single women, not well known to the doctor, complained of feeling tired and unwell. He got her to enlarge on this, and learnt that she had felt sluggish and cold lately. He took a full history and examined her, bearing in mind such possibilities as myxoedema and anaemia, which occurred to him early in the interview. He found nothing on examination, but sent her for appropriate tests.

2. *Detective type of personal interview*

The tests were all normal, but she still felt ill, so he asked her to come for a longer interview. He asked various questions about her life, and learnt that a recent change in the office had upset her. She was not easy to talk with, but he got a past history of a dominating mother, who rather isolated her, but made her feel she

33

should take a pride in her job, but that she would achieve little. She was now lonely and frustrated, and her symptoms dated from the office change which exposed her to a new and larger group of people who seemed unfriendly. He summarized this picture for her, as far as it went, and she agreed it was relevant to her symptoms and was grateful, so she said, for his interest. But at the same time she made the doctor feel that further questioning on these lines would meet resistance. He could never change her or her life situation. So he prescribed anti-depressants and asked her to return in a fortnight.

3. *Flash type of interview*

She returned even more depressed, and the doctor said 'Oh dear, we must try again' apologetically, at which she burst into tears. The doctor's immediate reaction was that she looked ridiculous crying in the hat she was wearing. This thought shocked him, since he likes to think of himself as sympathetic to his patients, but he realized at once that she might be making other people unsympathetic to her in a similar way. She started apologizing for her tears, and was surprised when the doctor apologized in turn for not letting her feel she could cry with him before. She felt at once the new relationship that this interchange had established, and understood what the doctor meant when he suggested that she might have been keeping people at arms' length by a rather stern manner. He referred to the hat, which was a formidable affair, and she took this point with interest and good humour. Finally she was able to agree that her initial complaint of feeling the cold might be because there was nobody to warm her up, but her stern manner was hiding this need from other people.

The first interview was 'illness orientated', with the doctor very reasonably looking for myxoedema, anaemia, or other physical illness.

The second interview was 'patient orientated', in a detective way. The doctor organized the interview to try to make a diagnosis of the patient herself rather than of an illness. He was aware of her as a cold dominating person, but was not involved very much with her himself.

The third interview was also 'patient orientated' but involved the doctor/patient relationship as well as the patient. The doctor had a flash of understanding and was able to share it with the patient. Before this could happen they both lowered the barriers, the doctor admitting his failure, and the patient letting herself cry. The interview was much warmer than the earlier ones and established a new relationship between doctor and patient, which should be useful in itself but also in helping her to react differently with other people.

THE 'DETECTIVE' TYPE OF TECHNIQUE

This is too well-known to need much description. The doctor may realize that he should explore a particular patient's problems which lie behind the illness presented. He uses the same sort of technique as a medical history taking and enquires about the patent's feelings and relationships, present and past, and observes the patient's answers and evasions and reactions. This often leads to a long interview and perhaps several further ones as well. The doctor will make some sort of diagnosis and use this to interpret things to the patient. He will be aware of the emotions aroused both in the patient and himself and be aware of the type of doctor/patient relationship that develops and will try to use this in treatment, but both the emotions and the interviews themselves will be under the doctor's control. As the case develops the doctor will decide which factors to concentrate upon.

Examples of Detective work

(1) *Mrs Ingham—Dr Silver.* A married woman, aged twenty-nine, came with her fourteen-month-old girl. At this initial interview she complained of bouts of depression and quarrelling with her husband, an antique dealer. She used to live in South Africa with her mother and she had been planning to return there with her husband. However the mother had died just at the time of their marriage four years previously, and they had changed their plans and stayed in England. The doctor got all this information by appropriate prompting, and he went on to gather more intimate facts. Her parents had divorced when she was seven and she had

35

lived with her mother and often quarrelled with her. The doctor suggested that perhaps she felt guilty over her mother. She agreed but became a bit tearful and withdrew from the doctor when he asked further about mother's death. He gave her tranquillizers and asked her to return in a week.

At the second interview she looked better, had stopped the tranquillizers herself. This was a long interview, and she talked of her husband. Their relationship was going through some difficulties. He had been building up his antique business. Previously she had been helping him in his work, but now she was looking after the baby. She talked of their marital rows. At the end of the interview the doctor brought her back to the previous subject saying: 'Perhaps next time we should discuss your mother'.

She tried to avoid the next interview, complained of indigestion and suggested that the doctor might talk to her husband, but with patience the doctor led her back to talking of the rows with her mother.

At the next two interviews she was better again. She had been talking to her husband and told the doctor a lot about her mother. Both she and her mother were strong-minded competent people who clashed at times, and the mother blamed her for the failure of a property deal which had been designed to enable them to live together. Gradually the doctor enabled her to unload to him the guilt and anger over these quarrels, and it was clear that she was reacting to the present situation with her husband in a similar way. At later interviews the doctor helped her to see that she had been treating men as rivals, and she was able to accept her role as wife and mother more contentedly.

This was a series of fairly short interviews, but the technique resembled one or two long interviews with useful pauses for the patient to ponder things and overcome her resistances.

The doctor focussed on the mother/husband aspects and controlled the case with this in mind. Presumably he could have reached a similar result from some other focus, but he stuck to what he saw, and it worked. When the emotive subject of her mother's death became too much for her she was allowed to escape and recover before going on. There must have been a good relationship holding doctor and patient together here, but successful though this 'detective' case was, we do not know what doctor and patient were feeling about each other, and like many focal detective cases, it was not discussed between them or used in the treatment explicitly.

(2) *Miss Malton—Dr Silver*. A single girl, aged thirty-one, complained of anxiety and depression. The employers for whom she worked were splitting up and reorganizing the firm. She was not sure of her position and was surprised to feel so upset about it. She mentioned that she had felt like this once before, when she had had a miscarriage, and here she started crying. The doctor tried to encourage her and sympathize with her. She told him that she would have loved to have a baby then, but it would have been quite impossible at that time. The doctor looked for a parallel between the present situation with the employers and the previous miscarriage, and suggested that perhaps on both occasions men had left her in a mess. She seemed rather distraught at this turn in the interview and the doctor gave her some sedatives and asked her to return in a week's time. She never came back. The mistake here was that the doctor was too quick to try to organize the case along his own line of thought. Things seemed to be going all right until he tried to add it up and test out his ideas with her. If he had not been in any hurry he could have let her express herself in her own way, instead of framing questions on a rather hasty assumption. The doctor's own enthusiasm and hasty interpretation had scared her off. Perhaps the doctor himself had become yet another man who was leaving her in a 'mess'.

(3) *Mr Quorn—Dr Sage*. This was a man aged forty-seven, on the doctor's list for fourteen years, but in fact he was a complete stranger to the doctor.

He came for a certificate to help him to change his job to something more conveniently near his home and he seemed depressed. The doctor enquired about his life, and got a brief outline with a few questions. Amongst other things he learnt that he had an adolescent son, and for a moment he nearly cried when he said that they could have no more children. This was because his wife had had puerperal psychosis after her son was born.

The doctor guessed that there might be some trouble with the adolescent son which had caused the present upset, but he felt he had made a good start and established a useful relationship with the patient, and he stopped there with a prescription for anti-depressants.

When we discussed the case in the seminar it became clear that the impetus for the interview came from the doctor's initial surprise at the patient's curious request, and also the fact that he had been on the list for a long time but was a stranger to him. He was framing questions with this in mind rather than letting the patient have the reins. Though he recognized the depression and guessed the cause, he didn't get the patient to express his distress when he saw the tears welling up, but rather covered it up by giving tablets instead.

The doctor felt satisfied that he had made a good start, but the patient evidently didn't share this feeling at the interview. He came back but somehow they could not work together.

However this case had an interesting and unexpected sequel. Eventually the patient sent his wife who disclosed she had been frigid lately. Her adolescent son had reminded her of her own brother, roused incestuous fears and put her off intercourse with her husband. The doctor was able to help her over this, and thereby the whole family benefited.

THE FLASH

These brief examples show how 'detective' work, with more formal questioning of the patient, and with the doctor keeping control of the case as it develops, can be very valuable if we are prepared to spend the time on the case. It cannot, however, be fitted so easily into the average ten-minute interview, though something of this sort must often be attempted if we are to understand our patients.

However if a flash occurs, this can transform the case. It may occur at any time during short or longer interviews, and it consists of a spontaneous mutual awareness of something important to the patient. We have found it easy to recognize a flash but more difficult to define it. It varies enormously with each doctor and patient and it is to some extent a part of ordinary human experience. In fact in the surgery we all frequently miss such possible interactions which could be valuable.

The doctor has to allow himself the discomfort of abandoning his own ideas of what should be happening and 'tune in' to the patient's distress. Often the flash concerns the relationship between doctor and patient, but even if it does not, the relationship is changed by the flash.

Examples of Flash technique

(1) *Mrs Fareham—Dr Gold.* This was a thirty-four-year old woman whose eldest child had died of congenital heart disease at the age of six weeks. She had two others aged four and two-and-a-half. She kept bringing the children to the doctor with minor ill-nesses and complaining that they would not sleep or were difficult, and often made aggressive jokes about them: 'You take them doctor,' and so on. The doctor knew well that Mrs Fareham was irritable and unhappy over them.

On this occasion she came with the youngest child who was said to have runny nose and eyes. The doctor could see nothing wrong and was rather at a loss. He was struck by the absence of Mark, the four-year-old, and he said 'Where's Mark?' She replied that he had just gone to school for the first time five days ago, and there was an immediate flash of understanding between them that this was really why she had come and what they had to discuss. The doctor let her talk and she was able to tell him, in front of the youngest child, how awful it had been for her, as well as the boy, to separate at the school, even though he was such a 'terror'. She said though it was silly, she feared something awful would happen to him at school. The doctor asked her to return in two weeks. When she did so she poured out her guilt over Mark, his behaviour was uncontrollable, she was frightened of hitting him sometimes and had sent him to school earlier than usual to get rid of him. With very little help she went on to talk about her self-blame over the deformity and death of her first child. In several successive interviews during normal GP contacts, she told the doctor of her feelings of being a bad mother and about the family squabbles. These have gradually lessened and the family tension is easier. The children are presented with less minor illnesses. The patient's husband came with a minor illness and reported how the family were much happier now.

It does not sound as though the doctor had done much or gone very deep in this case, but it seems clear that the whole family have been helped over a difficult stage. By the remark 'Where's Mark?' and her reaction to it, and the fact that they both recognized the importance of it, a much more honest doctor/patient relationship was allowed to develop. She was able to express and deal with the bad feelings inside her, instead of expressing them indirectly through presenting the children with minor illnesses, or with actually hitting them about. As she said herself, 'You see, if I didn't say that I might do something awful'.

(2) *Mrs Carlisle—Dr Black.* A married woman aged thirty-eight with three children. The doctor had previously made several attempts to understand this woman, who complained of tension headaches, was often distressed and anxious during contacts with the doctor for herself or family illnesses. The doctor had tried to get her to come back and discuss things several times, but she resisted this 'detective' approach. At this interview the doctor was aware of something different in her, perhaps a flirtatious look? He felt he really didn't understand her at all, possibly her husband didn't too. He said, 'Somehow I feel your husband and I are missing what you really want'. She immediately responded to this honest remark and said, 'It's funny you should say that, I've been working for some men who run a flower shop and one of them has been paying me attention lately'. Apparently this had aroused vague romantic feelings in her. She had told her husband, who made her stop working for them. The doctor then said, 'Would you like to come back and discuss it when I've got more time?' and she replied, 'No, I'll drop in and see you in two weeks perhaps'. The doctor then said, 'So it seems I must pay you enough attention but not too much'. She smiled at this and agreed. This was the flash.

She returned much more freely after this and kept up a rather teasing flirtatious sort of relationship with the doctor, who skilfully avoided either letting her take charge or doing so too powerfully himself. She talked of her husband in a rather derogatory way, saying 'men are funny', including the doctor here too. The doctor pointed out how she seemed to be enjoying making her husband look small, though this didn't help her much. At the next interview she said 'I've been thinking it over, you are right, my husband and I have been having an argument without words'. Gradually she realized how she felt about him, how unsure she was about herself, and how she must work things out for herself.

This patient is on the defensive, attacks the doctor and her husband to hide the poor opinion she has of herself. She would not allow a more formal approach by the doctor, still less would she tolerate going to a psychiatrist. However the doctor got through to her in the interview, as it happened putting himself in the husband's position and skilfully staying there while she reached more understanding about herself. There is no detective questioning here no diagnosis other than what is clear from the doctor/patient relationship itself, and what the doctor knows of her from the past. On the occasion of the flash she came in looking flirtatious, which was new. The doctor was somehow liberated from his traditional approach too and 'tuned in' to her need for a relationship which must not be too close. He actually established this relationship with her, explicitly, in the interview, not without some anxieties on both sides. She was later able to use this relationship to help her understand her marriage and relationship to other people in general. She is not in any sense a new woman as a result of this, but a small improvement in understanding herself in this way is worthwhile and a more realistic goal than a 'cure'.

(3) *Mrs Derby—Dr Sage.* A housewife, aged fifty-six, with no children. She has a sister living with her, and also her old father who recently came down from the north after his wife died. This old father had a tendency to be a 'grand invalid' and retire to bed, which the doctor had resisted. The patient came complaining of feeling faint and of a boil in the ear. While the doctor was dealing with this, she talked about her life with her father.

All GPs are familiar with this situation, where the patient has something other than the presenting complaint which they cannot quite tell us.

We are often uneasy here too, not sure whether to be the traditional doctor or to tune in to what the patient is saying. There may be many· reasons for stopping the patient's flow of talk and following our own line of thought. For example anxiety not to miss physical illness of importance, lack of time, or lack of sympathy. However this uneasiness, if we can tolerate it, is often the prelude to a useful flash. In this case the patient said of her father, 'He looks so weak when he gets up in the mornings, and I think ... another day to get through'. The doctor suddenly got the feeling that she was really talking about herself as well as her father. She agreed, and at once was on a new level with the doctor, talking of her own sadness and lack of children. She ended with, 'I wonder what will happen to me when I'm old and the only one left'. The doctor replied, 'I don't think your father is as sad as you are.'

Later the old father had a coronary, and as he recovered the patient retired to bed with a hip pain of no very clear nature. The doctor was able to say to her, 'Well you've managed it, you are having a rest now,' without giving offence and she was soon up again.

On another occasion she came complaining of faintness and tingling and seemed depressed again.

She talked of her father and sister and said 'My sister looks so like my mother, I think that's why father likes her so much'. The doctor helped her to express the jealousy behind the remark.

This depressed, rather ugly sister, competing for her father's affection, is gradually developing an intimacy with the doctor, who can understand her loneliness. She is aware of his concern, but finds it difficult to show much emotion and has to keep herself and others in control. The case continues and the doctor will be ready to help in a crisis such as the father's death.

The GP meets his patients and their families in apparently disconnected incidents over long periods. This gives ample opportunity for getting to know them, even without formal questioning or consciously summarizing the information, and it is in this setting that a flash is so valuable.

In the detective interview the doctor is behaving in the traditional medical role of diagnostic inquisitor. For a flash to occur, he usually has to abandon such traditional behaviour and tune in to the patient. Thus both doctor and patient lower their defences prior to a flash (e.g. Mrs Carlisle above 'I don't understand what you really want') and, though they tend to retreat to safer positions afterwards, the doctor/patient relationship is changed by the flash and this understanding is used by the patient. Though the doctor is less concerned with organizing the case and adding it up, he must still keep some control for the flash to be therapeutic.

For example, in the case Carlisle quoted above there is a danger that the doctor and patient might both get stuck in the relationship characterized by the phrase 'enough attention but not too much'. This is her usual pattern, and it would be easy for them both to collude in this and allow the relationship to go stale. The doctor must help her to understand and escape from this pattern of behaviour as far as is possible while the flash is still active in her mind.

Another difficulty for the doctor here is not to be blinded by his own flash, as it were, and to allow himself to retune to something else with the patient when this becomes appropriate. This is shown in the case Derby, where the doctor's habit of alert attention to what the patient brings has enabled them to deal with different aspects of her unhappiness at the moments when the tensions were ripe for this.

E

CHAPTER 5

The Development of the Form

M. J. F. COURTENAY

The usual method of presenting cases in seminars was to allow the doctor to report the case in his own style, with complete freedom to judge which aspects of the case were relevant, and to stress any part of the communication as he pleased.

This had two advantages; firstly, the most important moments of the contact were highlighted and secondly, the doctor's attitude towards the seminar was seen to reflect the patient's attitude towards the reporting doctor, *experienced directly by the seminar.*

There were however some disadvantages. In the first place negative findings were easily ignored and certain areas of the patient's functioning might not be studied at all. Secondly, it was a very time-consuming method of reporting.

This led to the attempts to produce a more formal presentation which, while avoiding the disadvantages, at the same time lost the advantages. This loss could only be offset by assuming that every doctor had an approximately equal skill and degree of sophistication in assessing what had occurred in the doctor/patient transaction. In previous research groups it had emerged that meaningful results could only be obtained by a more disciplined approach; the seminar therefore decided to structure their reports in terms of a 'Form'.

THE INITIAL INTERVIEW FORM

Initial Interview Forms have been developed for recording a long-interview over a number of years. They were introduced by

Michael and Enid Balint for the use of the case-workers in the Family Discussion Bureau[1] with the purpose of categorizing the information gained at an unstructured interview under various headings, so that both the positive and negative findings would appear with greater clarity and so allow an earlier and better diagnosis to be made.

This original Form was developed by the Focal Therapy Workshop, and the new one was then adapted for more general use at the Cassel Hospital. It was yet further modified for use by doctors working for the Family Planning Association during the course of a research seminar into the treatment of psycho-sexual disorders. The history of these forms has been dealt with elsewhere by M. Courtenay (1968).

However they were not designed to be used in the brief interviews which constitute normal general practice although Enid Balint, while leading a Research Seminar for General Practitioners, developed a Card to record cases presented in the seminar, the headings of which were similar to those used on the Forms (see Appendix 'A').

At the beginning of the present research project the seminar was faced with reporting interviews 'during which they thought that they had succeeded in making a meaningful contact with the patient and, using this, they had achieved something acceptable, provided that the interview did not last longer than ten to fifteen minutes' (see Chapter 1). It seemed likely that a greater understanding of the doctor/patient transaction in a brief interview might be gained by reporting it on a Form, especially as the headings on the Card used in the general practitioner seminar mentioned above were already available. However, it cannot be overstressed that the presentation on a Form of brief interviews occurring in general practice is very different from the process as applied to long-interviews. Firstly, the material recorded did not originate entirely within the key interview but included everything that the doctor previously knew about the patient and his surroundings and, in practice at any rate, a good deal of afterthought by the doctor concerned. Secondly, because the amount of material gained at a single contact

[1] Now known as the Institute for Marital Studies.

with regard to the doctor/patient relationship and its impact on the patient's disorder was always of a short, and even fleeting, nature, there was a great temptation to insert fantasies when facts were absent. Presenting a long-interview on a form is an exercise of organization and condensation, while presenting a brief interview often became like enlarging a photographic negative with a 'coarse-grain', so that when the magnified image appeared indistinct the doctor was inclined to retouch the final print. It must be said that the individual doctor was under great pressure from the group to do this, as any blanks in the report tended to be criticized severely, in spite of Michael Balint's reiteration that it was just these lacunae which should be observed and understood.

The Form developed rapidly during the first year of the seminar and then changed more slowly, finally reaching its definitive form during the fourth year. A summary of the headings and their development is set out in Table I.

TABLE I THE INITIAL INTERVIEW FORM

Mark: Heading:	I	II	III	IV	V	VI	VII	VIII	IX
(1) Factual material	*								)
(2) Presenting complaint & traditional diagnosis	*								)
(3) Overall diagnosis									
(a) Iatrogenous	*								)
(b) Autogenous	*				)				
(4) Therapeutic decisions									
(a) Traditional	*								)
(b) Focal	*		)						
(c) Overall	*								)
(5) Predictions	*								)
(6) Why case chosen					*	)			
(7) Patient's reactions			*						)
(8) Reasons for coming	*						)		
(9) Afterthoughts						*			)
(10) What patient wanted								*	)
(11) Collusion								*	)
(12) The Flash									*)

Perhaps the easiest way to understand the application of the formal approach is by illustration.

Mr Dalston, a young married man of twenty-five, presented complaining that he was becoming so fat that he seemed to be developing breasts. Some years previously he had suddenly put on a lot of weight and had developed striae on the upper arms and thighs. This had led to his admission to hospital to exclude the possibility of Cushing's disease, which was not confirmed. This episode occurred soon after the death of his grandmother, of whom he had been very fond. He had been married for a year to a girl who had been the reporting doctor's patient since childhood and who had an illegitimate baby which had died just before they had decided to marry. The doctor took up his anxiety about growing breasts, and it emerged that he had suffered from loss of libido, which he blamed on his wife's loss of interest and a generally unhappy atmosphere in the home. It also transpired that the baby who had died was not his. The doctor diagnosed the root of the problem to be concerned with anxiety about potency and focused on this.

It should be easy to accept that this brief account is a fairly accurate description of a fairly typical doctor/patient contact in the general practice setting. When reported in terms of the Form, however, it takes on altogether a more massive aspect, which serves, however, to clarify the various issues that pass rapidly and often almost unnoticed in a busy surgery. The case in formal terms reads:

Factual Material
Reporting Doctor: **Dr Black**
Patient's Name: **Mr Dalston**
Date of birth: 12-7-41 (aged 25)
Occupation: **Electrician**
Length of marriage: 1 year
Spouse's Name: **Brenda**
Date of birth: 20-8-44 (aged 22)
Occupation: **Clerk**
Children's Names: None living, but wife's illegitimate baby died of pneumonia August 1965 aetat 5/12

47

Six Minutes for the Patient

Date and Length of Interview: 24-2-67—15 minutes.
Length of time on doctor's list: 4 months.
Number of contacts: 3.
  Wife on list since 1953—75 contacts in 15 years (5 per year).

When and why the decision to report the case was made
When patient related previous episode of disturbance with previous stress (towards end of interview).

Presenting Complaint
Putting on too much weight again.
Traditional Diagnosis
Obesity.

Reasons for coming:
(a) *What the patient said*
    Came because growing a pair of breasts.

(b) *What the doctor thought*
    In trouble with his marriage.

Information Leading to Overall Diagnosis
Known previously
This was the patient's first contact with the doctor, though he had been seen by his partner a week previously with a cough and cold. There was a sheaf of letters from hospital, however, which the doctor read through when the patient related that he had been admitted for investigations of sudden obesity and skin striae. The letters referred to recurrent bronchitis in childhood, though the fact that he was overweight at the age of 15 was noted in passing. He was seen at hospital in 1962 with a story of having gained 2 stone 18 months previously, and was admitted to exclude Cushing's disease. He was 15 stone on admission, and lost the 2 stone by dieting quite quickly. He had courted a girl who had been a patient of the doctor's since he started practising in her area. She had had an illegitimate baby. The patient married her after the baby's death. She had had chorea as a child. Her mother had had 2 valvotomies for mitral stenosis. Her elder brother was sent to Borstal but has settled down. She has a step-father.

48

From observations made during this interview
The patient initially presented his weight increase, and then made special reference to his breast development and his striae, and referred at that time to the previous hospital admission. He then brought up the fact that he had loss of libido, in that he had intercourse less than once a week now, whereas before he had it two or three times a week. He thought this was partly due to the fact that his wife was not very keen on intercourse. He then went on to say that they were having frequent rows arising out of the wife saying he was idle in the home and did not decorate it like her friend's husbands (he admitted he was not much of a hand at this), while he complained of her being a spendthrift, always wanting to go out to expensive evenings dinner-dancing, etc., while he preferred pubs. He thought she had married him when she needed comfort after the baby died and was now regretting it. The doctor had not realized that the baby was not his until this interview; the wife had attended his partner at the time, and although the notes clearly stated that she had chucked the man who impregnated her, the doctor hadn't previously appreciated this fact. The patient had courted her while she was pregnant. The striae appeared as previously described in the hospital report. The breasts were fat but there was no evidence of any increase in nipple size or of glandular tissue. The doctor suggested that he must feel pretty miserable in the present atmosphere of marital discord, feeling that his wife was demanding money and work and refusing him love, and as thirst was often due to being upset, perhaps the over-eating was due to his being in a state. The remarks about growing breasts were interpreted as a fear of becoming less of a man and related to his reduction of libido. It emerged his wife wanted another baby now, but he felt she disliked his fat body.

Overall Diagnosis
(a) *Iatrogenous*: A man who had courted a girl impregnated by another man and was accepted during her bereavement, was now being rejected by her and was trying to comfort himself by eating and drinking, only to find this was making him less manly and attractive; leading to a vicious circle.

49

(b) *Autogenous*: Felt that he must be suffering from glandular trouble (? trouble with his testes) after all, in spite of the previous hospital reassurance.

Therapeutic decisions based on Traditional Diagnosis
1200 calorie diet.

Therapeutic decisions based on Overall Diagnosis
For this visit: To relate his obesity to his life situation.
For the future: To explore his anxieties about his potency.

Patient's reactions as observed during interview
Accepted the interpretation about eating and drinking to comfort himself and then told the doctor that he put on the 2 stone in weight after his grandmother, to whom he was very much attached, had died, concluding that that must have been why he had to eat so much then. He rejected the interpretation about becoming less of a man by saying he wasn't afraid of changing sex.

Afterthoughts while writing-up
None.

Predictions
(a) *Short-term*: Has achieved understanding with doctor and will be able to lose weight by dieting, but may then feel more under pressure in the marriage. ? production of new symptoms.
(b) *Long-term*: Depends on the severity of his sexual disturbance, not yet fully diagnosed.

This illustrative case was presented on the Form as it had been used during the first year of the research, and was little changed from the original Mark I Form developed from the old Record Card of a previous group.

The developments from this point may easily be presented in terms of the illustrative case. Firstly, it is clear that there is no provision for recording how the patient reacted to the doctor's therapeutic attempt, and this makes the whole report more doctor-centred than it should be. Secondly, the decision as to when and why the case was chosen was simplified to just 'why' and later abandoned altogether, because it became increasingly clear that this, too, was a function of the doctor rather than the patient. The discovery of the importance of the patient's contribution was perhaps the outstanding change of attitude by the members of the seminar during the project, even though the original Form included autogenous components both with regard to the reasons for coming and in the overall diagnosis itself. Experience with the reporting showed, however, that what was reported was often not the patient's fantasies but the doctor's fantasies about them! In the case of Mr Dalston the doctor had thought the patient was worried about his potency, whereas the seminar was convinced that the patient's orientation was strongly homosexual, and far from wanting to be made potent he was trying to get understanding from the doctor about this orientation.

Thirdly, there was a change in the headings concerned with the therapeutic decisions based on the overall diagnosis. Originally, and incidentally before the time that Mr Dalston was reported, these were couched in terms of a focal area, with points for and against considered at the same time. The focus was of necessity an intelligent guess that, in a brief interview, the doctor could hardly be expected to deal with the whole disturbance, but would have to choose an area most accessible to change and most likely to lead to a useful objective. After all, this approach had already yielded dividends in the Focal Therapy Workshop and the FPA Seminar on Psycho-sexual Problems.

What was not originally obvious was that in the long interview there is an opportunity to explore the whole personality and to allow a focus to crystallize out of the material. In the brief interview it is more a matter of chance whether a focus appears, though such a focus sometimes emerged as an afterthought. By the time Mr Dalston was presented the headings had been simplified by generalizing the therapeutic decisions into merely short-term and long-term plans. This case does not illustrate afterthoughts well either, because the doctor had made up his mind firmly, wrongly as it transpired.

It must be said that it was astonishing how much of the past history could be forgotten by the doctor during any given interview. One doctor had forgotten that a particular patient had been married twice, even though he had initiated sub-fertility investigations during her first marriage! In addition the full implications of the doctor's responses to the patient were often not fully appreciated until after the end of the interview, often not until the time to write the case up for presentation was reached.

All this led towards the realization that the Form should pay much greater attention to everything the patient contributed, either openly or unconsciously, and this led to a new series of headings which attempted to clarify the patient/doctor exchange. They were grouped as a check-list under a summary of the interview. At the same time the previously known information leading to the overall diagnosis became more distinct from the material arising at the key interview.

Initially greater emphasis had been placed on what the doctor had tried to get from the patient, rather than the other way round. For instance, Mrs Chester, a widow of sixty-nine, had recently lost her husband who had suffered a myocardial infarct while she was out of the house. She had felt guilty at not being with him at the time of his attack and sought reassurance that nothing could have been done to save him if she had not been out. This was given and accepted on a superficial level, but when the doctor tried to probe a little deeper into her feelings of guilt about her husband, he was rebuffed aggressively, and so had to accept the limitation imposed.

The pursuing by patients of their own ends was sometimes seen to lead to collusion by the doctor, as in the case of Mrs Olney. She was a Spanish widow with two children, living less than a mile from the doctor's surgery, who asked him to visit her on the pretext of some minor leg trouble, but was really anxious to obtain a travel allowance to enable her to visit her ailing mother at home. It transpired in seminar discussion that the doctor had obviously been reluctant to disclose that this helpless woman was entirely supported by the state. Her 'guilt' about asking for help never seemed to inhibit her from making constant demands, and this seemed linked with her experience of deprivation in childhood.

In this case it appeared that the collusion was that Mrs Olney should continue to be seen as a helpless foreign widow, while the doctor appeared as omnipotent, able to meet her needs whenever she cried for help.

These two points were both added to the check-list concerning the summary of the interview and were found to displace the need to have a heading concerning the reasons for the patient coming to the doctor, which was subsequently dropped. This underlines the fact that even the realization of collusive attitudes was by no means necessarily a negative issue, as the nature of the communication between doctor and patient during the ordinary general practice contact was becoming gradually clearer. It was at this point the need for a dynamic summary of the interview became obvious.

The evolution of the Form to this point paved the way to directing a very concentrated and receptive attentiveness on as much as possible of what really went on in the brief interview. Sudden insights, sometimes by the patient, often by the doctor, and latterly by patient and doctor at one and the same time lead to the description of the flash described in Chapter 1, 2, 3 and 4, the inclusion of which as the last of the check-list sub-headings completed the definitive Mark IX Form (see Appendix 'A').

THE FOLLOW-UP FORM

The apparent similarity of the Follow-up Form to the Initial Report Form is a snare and delusion. Follow-up Forms were devised for the Focal Therapy Workshop and the Family Planning Association Seminar but both tended to be badly filled in. This was because doctors accustomed to using Initial Report Forms naturally tried to use the Follow-up Forms in a similar way, with the result that a summary of a number (sometimes a large number) of interviews was condensed, and this was both more difficult and more frustrating than reporting the material gained at the initial (one, two or three) interviews.

What is difficult to appreciate is that the Initial Interview Form is describing a relatively static situation in which the doctor is attempting a diagnosis formulated in special terms; while the Follow-up Form is describing a dynamic situation over a period of time and attempting to keep track of how far this development followed from the original formulation of the case.

The previous history of Follow-up Forms is not as well documented as the Initial Interview Forms. Again it will be sufficient to start with the Card used by Enid Balint's Seminar

(Appendix 'A') which was the immediate precursor to the Mark I Follow-up Form used in the present research (which was also designed by Enid Balint). Although the main body of the Form was only adapted in detail, there was one important new heading referring to 'the correctness of the predictions', and secondly the 'material emerging from the seminar discussion' was made a separate heading in its own right. The Overall Diagnosis followed the Initial Interview Form's subdivisions. Changes in Predictions (Prognosis) was omitted at first but soon re-instated.

This is how a follow-up report of Mr Dalston appears on the Form:

Factual Material
Reporting doctor: Black
Name of patient and number of original report: Mr Dalston 48/2
Date previously discussed: 7-3-1967
Dates of subsequent interviews: 7-3-67, 10-3-67, 21-3-67, 11-7-67
Average length of interviews: about 10 minutes each.

New or changed Traditional Diagnosis
No change.

How far original predictions proved correct:
Short-term: incorrect—no loss of weight achieved.
Long-term: originally too vague—his marriage broke up soon afterwards.

New material pertaining to Overall Diagnosis
In general: Marital strife rapidly worsened, though the wife was pregnant. He remained passive, liking pub life. His wife accused him of liking his mates more than her. Felt he married for pity rather than love. He hates domination by women, he broke off a previous engagement because of this. The marital situation rapidly deteriorated and he left to return to his mother in July.

Comments on original information leading to Overall Diagnosis
The material pointed the way fairly clearly.

Changes and additions to the Overall Diagnosis
Patient's homosexual orientation emerged more clearly in successive interviews.

Changes in Predictions (in terms of doctor/patient relationship, symptomatology and patient's life situation)
Patient seems to have retired from both the marriage and the doctor. No further treatment opportunities would seem likely.

Summary of changes and additions following seminar discussion
A more complicated picture than Dr Black's emerged from the discussion; the patient's problem seemed to be not his potency but his desire to have another man's baby. Doctor and patient were thus inevitably at cross-purposes, and Dr Black, finding the homosexual overtones disquieting, ignored them. The patient has now withdrawn, whether permanently or not remains to be seen. He would find it difficult to admit either that he had got his wife pregnant, or that someone else had impregnated her. It was possible however that he would return once the baby was born.

Summary of comments on doctor's technique
Six interviews since report. Patient has now left wife and doctor. After the initial interview Dr Black could not get near this man. He has never got near the wife either.

He attempted to help him in the marriage situation and ignored his offers: 'I'm not afraid of changing sex,' or 'I prefer my mates'. The seminar felt he might have helped by making this the focus of the doctor/patient relationship. The patient could not stand being made more potent.

When the first year's cases were followed up a heading dealing with the discussion of the doctor's technique was seen to be necessary, as this was only touched on in the Initial Interview Form. This Form then became current for a considerable time. Changes were minor and were related to the changes produced by the evolution of the Initial Interview Form, though at one stage this became confusing in practice because it was difficult to keep pace with them.

Later a new heading was introduced concerning 'Changes in Therapeutic Decisions', and in addition the New Overall Diagnosis was given a separate heading to make it readily identifiable. However, this Follow-Up (FU) Form (Mark VIII) was so massive in appearance that the seminar rebelled, and a simplified version was attempted. Unfortunately the simplification, while allowing greater

55

freedom for the reporting doctor to present fresh material, led to
a loss of precision in the essential function of the FU Form, namely
to chart the progress of the doctor/patient contact in terms of the
original formulation.

When this became apparent the Mark XI Form was produced,
combining as much freedom as possible in the context of a formal
approach. Table II summarizes the evolution of the various headings throughout the development of the FU Form:

TABLE II THE FOLLOW-UP FORM

Mark: Heading:	*I II III IV V VI VII VIII IX X XI*
(1) Factual material	*———————————————————)
(2) New or changed trad- itional diagnosis	*————————————————)
(3) New material re Overall Diagnosis	*———————————————————)
(4) Changes in Overall Diagnosis	*———————————————————)
(5) Changes in Predictions	*———————————————————)
(6) Correctness of Predictions	*———————————————————)
(7) Changes & additions during discussion	*——————————( )————)
(8) Discussion of doctor's technique	*————————( )————)
(9) Changes in thera- peutic decisions	——*( )————)
(10) New Overall Diag- nosis	*———————
(11) Improvement rating	*———)

From the research point of view, follow-up is concerned principally with evaluation. In this research the main issues in follow-up
were the efficiency of the original diagnostic formulation in terms
of the Initial Interview Form, the doctors' technique, and whether
the objectives were attained. The second and third issues are dealt

with in Chapters 1, 2, 3, 4, 5, and 9, which only leaves the question of the formal presentation for the present chapter.

Apart from the temporary hiatus consequent on the Mark X Form allowing very free *reportage,* the seven main headings remained virtually constant. The two main innovations are seen to follow firstly, an appreciation that doctors are more unpredictable than patients so that a close watch on changes in the therapeutic decisions had to be kept; and secondly, the need for recording carefully the development of the overall diagnosis during further doctor/patient contacts. A new formulation was often obscured by the prominence of small additions relating to the original formulation made some considerable time previously.

These considerations really relate to the fundamental difficulty, mentioned at the start of this review of FU Forms, in adequately formulating a dynamic situation, in that it is difficult to be succinct in recording a developing entity.

In conclusion it may be said that the seminar found the Follow Up Forms more irksome to use than the Initial Interview Forms, probably because of this difficulty. Reports were sometimes either impossibly long-winded, or so condensed as to be almost meaningless. However, in spite of this they were used, and this in itself is remarkable.

CHAPTER 6

The Diagnosis

MAX B. CLYNE

The term 'diagnosis', derived from the Greek verb *diagignoskein* (to distinguish, discern), means 'determination of the nature of a diseased condition: identification of a disease' (The Shorter Oxford English Dictionary (1968)). Physicians have not always felt the need to identify disease; the books of the Hippocratic collection do so no more than in general, vague, and ill-defined terms (e.g. crisis, fever, apoplexy). The science of diagnostics was born when physiological and pathological processes began to understand in terms of the natural sciences. In the early days of scientific medicine the physician often was unable to do more for his patient than to establish an accurate diagnosis, as treatment for many disorders was signally lacking. The vastly greater extent and power of our therapeutic armoury has, on the one hand, increased the need for accurate and precise diagnoses in the traditional sense and, on the other, has diminished this need, because some of our modern therapeutic measures are so embracing that they will cure even though a diagnosis may not have been established.

THE TRADITIONAL DIAGNOSIS

The traditional diagnosis is meant to place the illness within a known framework and to structure it in terms common to both doctor and patient, but considerable misunderstandings may arise here. Boyle (1970) had studied the difference between patients' and doctors' interpretations of common descriptive (diagnostic) terms as used by patients and doctors. He had found that apparently simple expressions, e.g. 'flatulence', 'diarrhoea', 'constipation', 'heartburn', and terms of localization ('kidney region', 'heart region') had at times completely different meanings (both intellectually and emotionally) for the doctor and for the patient. And confusion of tongues is even more common when diagnoses proper are expounded. An incidental case report (not discussed in our seminar) will illustrate this: a patient of mine, a young woman, brought her child, a strapping boy of six years old, to my consulting room. I told her that the child was suffering from bronchitis. To my surprise she began to shed bitter tears of despair. To me 'bronchitis' in this context had meant a relatively harmless, acute, inflammatory affliction of the bronchi, quickly cured by antibiotics. To her it means a terrifying disease that years ago had strangled an aged relative towards whom she had had ambivalent feelings of loving and hating.

Making a diagnosis is thus not merely an intellectual exercise, but it also has emotional connotations for both patient and doctor. Even before the patient has consulted his doctor, he will have arrived —in an effort to allay and contain his anxiety—at some kind of home-made diagnosis, the content and terminology of which will depend upon his intellectual status, his medical knowledge and his fantasies. The diagnosis subsequently made by the doctor, if communicated to the patient, may further allay the patient's anxiety. It certainly serves the purpose of allaying the doctor's anxiety, in that the doctor will feel able to handle the situation better.

The object of making a traditional diagnosis is thus twofold. On the intellectual level it is an assessment of a patient's disease or disorder to indicate the etiology and the effect of the disease on structure and function, for the purposes of classification, prognostication and treatment. On the emotional level it serves to structure an anxiety-arousing situation, so that anxiety—both the patient's and the doctor's—may be allayed.

One might ask whether it is sufficient to assess the disease or disorder—whether it might not be as important to examine the healthy parts of the patient. One might also ask whether it is sufficient to assess solely the patient's condition, or whether it might not be as important to examine his relationship with others, or to include the people around him in the diagnostic assessment. One

F

might further ask whether and to what extent it is desirable, therapeutically useful, or justified to allay the patient's and the doctor's anxieties. The question also arises whether and to what extent traditional diagnoses do indeed achieve the above objectives. It might be easier to answer these questions with the aid of an illustrative case report:

Miss Malvern—Dr Green

Previous history: An unmarried woman, forty-one years old, who had a good secretarial job, had been attending her doctor and his partners for the last two years on account of her asthma, from which she had been suffering for many years. At times the attacks became so severe that she had to be treated with corticosteroids. One day she visited her doctor to tell him that she was having treatment from a private psychotherapist. She mentioned on this occasion her mother, whom she described as 'psychotic' and 'grasping'. When the patient was a child her mother had told her that she was ugly and that nobody would ever want her. Indeed, the patient had never married and said that she felt 'on the shelf'. She also complained of feeling depressed. The doctor spoke to the psychotherapist (a woman) on the telephone and learned that the patient's mother, sister, and aunts had been in and out of psychiatric hospitals. The psychotherapist told the doctor that in her opinion the patient wanted to be physically ill rather than feel mentally disturbed. She also suggested the doctor be optimistic about the outcome and treat the patient with as little medication as possible. For the next few weeks the doctor followed the pyscho-therapist's suggestions. He gave the patient a tranquilliser and a certificate to stay away from work, but did not examine her further. It turned out later that the patient had, in fact, been attending two psychotherapists, one being a man, the other a woman, who were in touch with each other regarding the patient.

The interview: Two months after the first interview the patient returned to the doctor. She was more wheezy and appeared disgruntled, apparently because the doctor had not continued with the previously given anti-asthmatic drug. The doctor said that he thought that she was angry with him. She agreed and smilingly said he was not doing much for her. She then began to complain to the doctor about her boss. He had installed in her office a copying machine that produced a great deal of heat and fumes. The doctor suggested that she should write to the boss and ask him to make different arrangements, and he gave her a certificate in support of such a letter. The doctor then said to her that both the boss and the doctor were not really such ogres as she felt them to be, but that they needed prodding sharply into sympathetic action on her behalf. This ended the interview. By then she had stopped wheezing.

Let us try to elicit a traditional diagnosis from the material of this brief case history. In traditional medical work the doctor's attention would from the beginning have been focussed on the wheezing, and this together with the patient's history and physical examination might have led to further investigations. In fact, five years before the last-mentioned interview a battery of allergy tests had been carried out, which had produced no evidence of any allergic cause of the wheezing. No obvious physical abnormalities had been discovered on examination. These are common findings in *bronchial asthma*, the traditional diagnosis of the case. A physician with a little more perspicuity might have added to the main diagnosis of 'bronchial asthma' the subsidiary diagnosis of 'depression'. Less discerning physicians might have shrugged off this subsidiary diagnosis, thinking that a woman who for years had been suffering from a suffocating disorder would obviously be depressed.

The brief traditional diagnosis, be it 'asthma' or 'asthma and depression', has at least achieved one of the objectives stated above; it has classified the disorder. It has, however, not indicated the etiology of the disease and its effect on structure and function, though this might be remedied. The traditional diagnosis might be extended to read: *Sporadic asthma of unknown, perhaps psychological origin, without structural effects on the respiratory tract, with X% loss of respiratory function (as determined by pneumometry); depression (perhaps reactive to the asthma), producing little, if any, loss of functioning.*

Six Minutes for the Patient

THE IMPLICATIONS OF THE TRADITIONAL DIAGNOSIS

What about the other aims (prognostication, treatment)? Taking a population of patients suffering from disorders that would be subsumed under our extended diagnosis, it might be possible to stipulate a probability that the patient would or would not recover (i.e. a prognosis). This could be done only in *statistical* terms, but not truly in predictive terms based on the actual condition of the particular patient. If, for argument's sake, it were known from previous investigations of a population of patients suffering from sporadic asthma of the kind described that, say 60% (with a standard deviation of $\pm 5\%$) had lost their asthma within five years, one would be able to foretell that our patient would be likely to recover from her asthma with a 60% $\pm 5\%$ probability within five years. It is not possible, however, to prognosticate on the basis of the traditional diagnosis that our particular patient would lose her asthma, say, provided she got married, or changed her job, or became less depressed. The traditional diagnosis will thus allow no more than a prognosis of statistical probability, but not a personal, unique prognosis.[1]

The same applies to treatment. Experience with other patients, either by scientific investigation or by the practical, remembered experience of the physician, will indicate a certain degree of statistical probability that certain treatments might improve or cure the condition. Again, the traditional diagnosis will not lead to any kind of personal, definitive treatment of any particular patient. In fact, on the basis of the traditional diagnosis, it is quite inexplicable that the patient's wheezing should have stopped at the end of the interview.

There are thus two major objections to confining the assessment of a patient's case to the traditional diagnosis: firstly, that it provides no specific and personal predictions and treatments of individual patients, especially not when emotional disorders or the emotional aspects of disease are concerned, and secondly, that the traditional diagnosis really describes, classifies and assesses an

---

[1] A leading article in the *Lancet* (1969) on the psychiatric diagnosis states that 'to expect prognostic validity is to expect too much of the (psychiatric) diagnosis'.

abstract concept, viz. the disease or illness, and not the sick person. It is apparently quite irrelevant in the context of the traditional diagnosis that our patient was unmarried at forty-one years of age, that she had treatment simultaneously both from her doctor and from two private psychotherapists, that she felt denigrated by her mother and 'on the shelf', that several members of her family, including her mother, had been mentally ill, that she had certain habitual images of and attitudes towards men in superior positions (her boss and her doctor). Some of these features, e.g. the fact that there was mental illness in her family, might possibly have been part of the traditional diagnosis ('heritable'). Others, e.g. her attitude to men, would certainly have been thought to be quite irrelevant by most physicians in the context of the traditional diagnosis.

The traditional diagnosis is concerned only with the pathological condition, in this case 'asthma'. It is an *illness-centred* diagnosis. This does not necessarily devalue it. The traditional illness-centred diagnosis has its merits, as otherwise it would hardly have survived in practical medicine for several centuries. It produces an excellent framework for the classification of disease and is invaluable for statistical and epidemiological purposes. It enables many diseases to be treated by highly specific means, and it may indicate the statistical probability of the outcome of certain diseases.

Yet, traditional diagnoses are certainly not the best or even true accounts of many patients' conditions, especially in general practice. So much more is known about patients, has made an impact during consultations, has been felt by the doctor—difficult though this may be to perceive and record—that most general practitioners consider the traditional diagnosis, as written into patients' clinical notes, to be no more than an aide-memoire. Daily experiences of inexplicable recoveries, failures, and syndrome-shifts are so common that in many cases the traditional diagnoses seem to be utterly off the target. Karl Menninger has written: 'Patients who today crowd the physicians' offices or fill the hospital beds suffer for the most part from conditions to which no single [i.e. traditional] label can be given'. The nagging feeling that our traditional diagnoses and the treatments and prognoses based on these diagnoses bear no relationship to the true circumstances of the patient's condition and to our work and its results, has brought many general practitioners to Dr Michael Balint's seminars.

Furthermore, in general practice patients are often treated (and well treated) without a traditional diagnosis either having been established or being appropriate to the kind of treatment being given. In fact, the patient is often at the greatest disadvantage from the point of view of health or survival when the traditional diagnosis is most refined. The best, most detailed and best founded diagnoses are usually presented at clinico-pathological conferences, when the patient is already dead. Traditional diagnosis also carries the danger that the patient and the doctor may use it (i.e. the structuring of the illness) as a defence against discovering the emotional conflicts that may underlie the patient's illness. To give another example from my own practice (not discussed in our seminar): A woman came to see me, unhappy, crying, because her husband had forced her to leave their flat and had put in for divorce. She told me quite convincingly that she intended to commit suicide. The traditional diagnosis would be 'reactive depression'. The treatment based on this diagnosis might have consisted of anti-depressant drugs, perhaps admission to psychiatric hospital. Judging by statistical results of these treatments the woman's symptom of depression would most likely have improved or disappeared. But her real problem and true illness was her aggressiveness towards men, which took the form of emotionally emasculating every man with whom she had any relationship. She was an expert in presenting herself as being helpless and in need of love and care, arousing men's protective urges, and then by increasing her demands making their fulfilment impossible, so that in the end the men in her life had felt that she was more than they could take and had deserted or rejected her. Whenever she lost the target of her demanding aggression she would turn her aggression guiltily towards herself and threaten or even attempt suicide.

The traditional diagnosis and the treatment arising from it would have structured and fortified her basic illness. 'Reactive depression' would have implied (in the doctor's mind as well as in the patient's) that the illness 'depression' was a reaction to what others (her husband, former boy-friends) were doing to her. Even with the symptom 'depression' cured, she would still have reacted compulsively to men as she did before—with the same consequences.

Balint (1959) has redefined the term diagnosis as denoting an 'understanding of people in a professional capacity'. In a study of night and emergency calls (Clyne, 1961) in which some members of our present research group participated, we confirmed that the traditional diagnosis was of little help in determining appropriate treatment in those situations. We felt that we needed a more embracing, deeper, or wider diagnosis that would enable us to formulate proper treatment plans. In our present study we felt this need even more, viz. to spell out and record a diagnostic assessment that would include those features of the patient's personality and relationships that delineated him within the various spheres of his life. It became one of our aims to present a diagnosis that would give an overview of the patient's physical and emotional condition and of his relationships with himself and others, including the doctor, a global or *overall diagnosis*, as we called it.

Let us return to the illustrative case report of the woman presenting with asthma. The overall diagnosis was stated by the reporting doctor as: 'Asthma, this being more comfortable than the problems it conceals, e.g. fear of being afflicted by familial mental illness; and difficulties relating to men'. This was extended during the discussions of the case to: 'The patient divides herself between her therapists, provoking rivalry and competition between them. She is creating confusion about the person who is really in charge of her case by presenting her emotional conflicts to her psychotherapists and her asthma to her general practitioner, but—at the same time—also presenting each with the problems that the other is supposed to deal with. She does the same to others with whom she has relationships out of fear of being left on the shelf. This feeling is a reflection of her mother's image of her as ugly and useless, though the doctor finds her an acceptable, attractive woman who looks younger than her age'. A year later the reporting doctor added that the patient's attacks used to recur whenever she was asked out by a man or when she was confronted by apparently insoluble difficulties. The asthma appeared to be a cry for help, a demand to her doctor to control her and yet allow her to be ill.

In contrast to the traditional diagnosis the overall diagnosis largely contains statements which refer to the patient's relationships, including that with her doctor, and to the specific anxieties which are connected with her symptoms and signs (perhaps causally, perhaps concomitantly). The overall diagnosis differs further from the traditional diagnosis in that the latter is more or less a static concept, whilst the overall diagnosis is ongoing in that it is varied or extended at each interview.

The overall diagnosis (assuming that it is indeed superior to the traditional diagnosis in so far as it will produce a better treatment plan and a more accurate prognosis) also scores over the traditional diagnosis in that it is a *patient-centred* diagnosis. It conveys a picture of a human being whose conflicts and sufferings can be felt and understood. In a sense it is tailormade: the doctor's actions are based no longer on statistical probabilities, but on the specific needs of the individual patient. The term 'patient-centred', when used in relation to our overall diagnosis, has often aroused animosity among colleagues with whom we have discussed our findings, because every doctor believes that he is centring his efforts on the individual patient and that all medical activities are *per se* patient-centred. The term is thus taken as a slur on doctors who use the traditional diagnosis and as an expression of hubris on the part of doctors of our way of thought.

Many doctors—both in general practice and in hospital—say that they are, in fact, establishing overall diagnoses in any case, although they may use the traditional diagnosis as a recording device. They may claim that their knowledge of the patient's background, their enquiries, the findings of social and psychiatric social workers, when employed, will supply any material that is relevant to the patient's condition and, although not stated in so many words in the diagnosis, will be used for the treatment plan and the prognosis. Undoubtedly, most if not all doctors feel the need for and are trying to use patient-centred medicine, but by tradition and clinical training are fettered to illness-centred medicine. The discomfiture often felt when illness-centred medicine and traditional diagnoses fail, be it on account of inexplicable turns of the disorder, of symptom-shifts, unexpected recoveries or deteriorations, is an expression of the cleft between clinical tradition and the doctor's intentions.

Probably in our case of the asthmatic woman many general practitioners—had she been their patient—would have been acquainted with some or even all of the data of the overall diagnosis. Yet this knowledge would most likely have remained outside readily recalled awareness, might have been treated as not truly relevant, or might have been seen as relating to factors which are not within the doctor's realm or which he cannot do anything about anyway. In any case, unless an overall diagnosis is properly formulated, it cannot be used as a rational basis for a treatment plan or a prognosis, except in the vaguest possible way. In fact, the details of relationships and feelings mentioned in the overall diagnosis of our patient Miss Malvern are hardly ever recorded or made use of.

THE IMPLICATIONS OF THE OVERALL DIAGNOSIS

The touchstone of the superiority of the overall diagnosis over the traditional diagnosis and of its usefulness and validity will be the accuracy with which it describes and assesses the patient and his illness and the extent to which it enables a detailed treatment plan and prognosis to be deduced from it.

Let us study the treatment plan stipulated by the doctor for Miss Malvern. After the initial interview he thought that he should concentrate on the anger she showed when she was with him and her boss, a course for which her resentment seemed to have left no alternative. He wanted to allow her to express her anger, to show that he could tolerate it and that she would be better for releasing it. He also wanted to prevent her from rendering him ineffectual, as he felt she was trying to do by dividing her problems neatly into those offered to his partners, to him, and to her psychotherapists. This was based on his feeling that she really needed him as somebody she could lean on.

The doctor presented a follow-up report three years after the initial interview and described the changes of the treatment plan during that time. The patient had meanwhile changed her job; she was training to become a social worker. She had experienced some difficulties with her instructors because she was trying to please each too much, and she had similar difficulties with her mother and boy-friend. Incidentally she had had no attacks of asthma for over two years. The doctor had been aiming to help her to become independent of her mother (in other words, to remove her need for having attacks of asthma), to help her to achieve a degree of sexual maturity (of which the acquisition of a boy-friend was a sign) and to help her in a paternal way to become more self-assured. He also decided not to communicate further with the psychotherapist.

In the discussion of the follow-up report another aim was added: to enable her to come to the doctor when her anger became too much for her, so that the doctor might help her to control this anger.

Were the treatment aims in the case of Miss Malvern derived from the overall diagnosis? Let me summarize the overall diagnosis: the patient had used her asthma as (1) an escape, (2) as a cry for help, (3) and as a demand to the doctor for control; further (4) she divided herself (her problems) between her helpers.

The doctor's plan to allow her to express her anger derived directly from (1), to gain independence from her mother from (2), to help her to control her anger from (3).

Had these treatment aims been fulfilled? From a further follow-up report a year later we learned that the patient had gone through a crisis situation. Her sister, to whom she was very close, had died, and she had experienced some stress at work, but she had had no more asthma. She had taken some steps towards gaining independence and more self-assurance, for she had been able to control her aggressive feelings with the help of the doctor. She also had made a success of her job. The doctor had not stipulated any specific aim as regards her sexual maturity, and, in fact, she had made very little progress towards it.

On the basis of the overall diagnosis the following predictions had been made: the particular kind of relationship between the patient and the doctor would continue for many years, and the asthma would diminish or disappear, provided that the doctor did not become more powerful than the patient would permit him to be. It was also predicted that she would not get married. These predictions were indeed fulfilled.

We felt in the course of our work that these agreements between overall diagnosis, treatment plan and its results, and predictions confirmed our assessment of the usefulness of the overall diagnosis. We applied the concept of the overall diagnosis to all our reported cases. Perhaps a few brief examples from our research cases will illustrate the type and spirit of these overall diagnoses:

Mrs Exton—Dr Sage

Traditional Diagnosis: Sinusitis and reactive depression.

Overall Diagnosis: A frightened and depressed mother, whose first child at two years of age was thought to have severe kidney disease. She has been over anxious ever since, and the marital relationship has become a casualty. Her aggression has been turned on herself, as her husband has turned his back on her.

Miss Exford—Dr Scarlet

Traditional Diagnosis: Wants pregnancy terminated, facial acne.

Overall Diagnosis: A girl with low self-esteem and handicapped by a faulty mother-daughter relationship. She recognizes her need for men to be concerned for her, but can form only shallow and short-lived relationships. These reinforce her feelings of femininity, but not sufficiently to make her confident enough to continue with her pregnancy. She is an unhappy girl, who is forcing people to treat her in an off-hand manner.

These overall diagnoses obviously were not totally unrelated to their respective traditional diagnoses. In the case of Mrs Exton the term 'depression' in the traditional diagnosis remains in the overall diagnosis and, furthermore, does imply 'aggression turned on herself' (in the overall diagnosis). The term 'reactive' in the traditional diagnosis implies some environmental stress related to the depression ('husband has turned his back on her' in the overall diagnosis).

ARRIVING AT AN OVERALL DIAGNOSIS

There is a further, methodological link between the traditional and the overall diagnoses. Traditionally medical men investigate by observation, taking a history, and examining, usually in that order. History taking, the central feature of medical investigation, is a highly standardized procedure, based on a schema from which questionnaires may be derived. We also used this procedure for our overall diagnoses. Obviously such statements as 'first child at two years of age was thought to have serious kidney disease' (Mrs Exton), 'a faulty mother-daughter relationship' (Miss Exford) arose out of a sort of history taking. Unless we already knew details of the patient's life history we asked questions and expected answers, especially if we wanted to present a case to the seminar and had to be prepared for a detailed cross-examination.

Here we found ourselves faced with a curious and disturbing contradiction. It was a maxim of our school of thought not to follow the traditional course of history-taking (i.e. asking the standard questions) but to observe the patient, to let him talk, and to 'listen' (in the sense in which Balint (1957) used this term). We knew only too well that questioning a patient about the facts of his life situation was not usually the best method of elucidating his feelings about those aspects of his life. Questions often put people on the defensive, and facts alone do not provide insight into human beings.

We often found it very difficult to formulate overall diagnoses even in successful cases, because our knowledge of the patient's total situation seemed scanty and patchy. The members of the seminar frequently pressed the reporting doctor to carry out further enquiries. The doctor then—often with reluctance—carried out a kind of inquisitional detective work in an effort to supply the factual material that the seminar thought necessary for a proper overall diagnosis. This needed long interviews at times, a technique that was not acceptable to some doctors and certainly not germane to our avowed aim of studying what went on in ordinary National Health Service general practices.

As we continued the studies of the case reports in our seminar a restless feeling developed among some members that the brief

70

The Diagnosis

general practice interview did not really lend itself to obtaining the overall view that would enable us to formulate a proper overall diagnosis and that more material seemed to be needed. The old argument of 'not enough time' came up. We were vexed, because we thought we had done good work in many cases with brief interviews, and we felt in our bones that the argument was really nugatory. It was even claimed by some sceptics in the seminar that the results of our research had shown that the overall and emotional aspects of a patient's illness could not be dealt with in the brief interviews of National Health Service general practice, because they supplied insufficient data for proper formulation.

THE FOCAL AREA IN THE OVERALL DIAGNOSIS

We came to the conclusion that extensive investigation of the global life experiences and situation of a patient was impracticable, even impossible, and was, in fact, not our normal procedure in our general practices. We thought, therefore, that what actually had happened in our successful cases and what we ought to do generally was to focus our attention on one particular aspect of the patient's world that seemed to be the major pathological domain. We called this the *focal area*, following the example of a group of workers (Malan (1963); Balint, Balint, Gosling and Hildebrand (1966)), who had developed the concept of a diagnostic and therapeutic focus in 'brief psychotherapy', a specific technique used by psychoanalysts. Perhaps another report taken from our research cases may illustrate this concept.

Mr Baldock—Dr Green

A man, forty-four years of age, came to ask the doctor for a National Health Insurance Certificate to return to work. The traditional diagnosis was: 'lumbar disc lesion'. The overall diagnosis as given by the doctor was: 'he has a sense of failure; he could have got a better job; he is homosexual, tied to his mother and female relatives; he is angry with his manipulating mother; he himself

71

manipulates the doctor. He wants a doctor who can tolerate his 'dirty' illnesses (he has had syphilis) and allow him to have stress illnesses instead, such as his backache'.

This is a fairly extensive overall diagnosis, which includes an understanding of the roots of the anxiety that had brought the patient to his doctor. It also assesses the disturbances of the relationships of the patient, the way in which he views his own role, the doctor's feelings for his patient, and some other aspects of the patient's total life situation:

(1) His failure at his job (work aspect).
(2) His homosexuality (sexuality aspect).
(3) His being tied to his female relatives and his being angry with his manipulating mother (family aspect).
(4) His manipulating the doctor, in that he wants a general practitioner who can tolerate him (doctor aspect).
(5) His desire or need to have stress illnesses, viz. his bad back (self respect).

Any of these aspects might be a focal area. In this particular case there had been no complaint against the reporting doctor about any paucity of knowledge about his patient. On the contrary, the overall diagnosis contained such a plenitude of information that obviously a need for selection arose both for the treatment plan and the predictions. Yet the discussion showed that members of the seminar were still not satisfied with this overall diagnosis. An unending number of questions was asked, such as: Is he actually homosexual or only in his fantasies? What does he do with his aggressive feelings? Is his physical illness an expression of self-destruction? The questions were all pertinent and relevant, yet they merely extended the overall diagnosis without making the choice of a focal area any easier.

Whether the overall diagnosis was to be accepted as it stood or whether it was to be supplemented by further enquiry, the major question now arose which particular area or aspect of this patient's life situation was to be investigated and treated. Should one deal with them all or several or one?

In fact the further we went into the question of defining and treating a focal area, the more we found ourselves in difficulties. In the case of Mr Baldock the doctor had determined his treatment plans by focussing on one particular aspect of the patient's illness. He thought that he should get the patient to acknowledge his sense of failure, and he predicted that the patient would let the doctor share with him his sense of failure, with therapeutic consequences. The predictions were, however, not fulfilled. We had similar disappointments in a number of cases because the focus seemed to change in subsequent interviews, either because other focal areas that had not been touched by the doctor gained in importance or because the focus had apparently been chosen inappropriately. In the case of Miss Malvern, the asthmatic woman, her aggressive feelings towards men in authority seemed at first to be the proper focal area. This was changed later to 'her rendering the doctor ineffective and compartmentalizing her problems', then to her relationship with her mother; her own self-assurance. and her sexuality. It seemed, not only in this but also in other cases, that these focal areas were chosen and changed at random, depending upon the patient's and the doctor's fancies.

In the case of Miss Malvern something had happened during the first interview to which the members of the seminar had paid only little attention. The doctor reported the interview as I have presented it. The subsequent discussion dealt almost exclusively with the features that we thought were of importance for our overall diagnosis: her psychotherapist, her mother, her feeling of being on the shelf, etc., whilst the central emotional event of the interview was not touched on: the doctor had told us that the patient appeared disgruntled, that he had felt her anger and that he had suggested to her that she was angry with him. She had agreed and with a smile had said that the doctor was not doing much for her. She then talked about her anger with her boss, who by installing a smelly office machine had increased her asthma. The doctor, with a sudden feeling of enlightenment and understanding, suggested that both the boss and he were not really such ogres but that both needed prodding into sympathetic action.

Only much later, in fact not until two years later, did we comprehend that this brief emotional interchange, which at the time of reporting appeared casual, introductory, and anecdotal, was really of great importance for the understanding of this and many other cases. On re-reading the transcripts of the seminar sessions concerned with Miss Malvern, the short shrift the seminar made of the emotional content of the initial interview is quite remarkable. Equally remarkable, the reporting doctor had in fact used the emotional content of the interview for his overall diagnosis and treatment plan, and had also used this emotional content as the basic material for the subsequent interviews, without at the time having been fully aware of its importance. Obviously the doctor at that time had perceived something in the patient which had struck a chord in him, and he was able to convey this understanding to her.

THE INTERRELATIONSHIP DIAGNOSIS

The study of many similar case reports made us realise that such mutual perceptions between doctor and patient did occur fairly frequently. They seemed to be the significant determinants of our diagnoses, treatments and prognoses; at least, we could see in retrospect that we had acted on them though we might not have been able to perceive them intellectually or put them into words at the time. This kind of interaction, the almost immediate understanding between doctor and patient, had the character of a flash of lightning. We called it therefore 'the flash'. The wider concept of the flash has been discussed in Chapters 1, 2 and 3. I am going to discuss here only the diagnostic implications of the flash.

In the case of Miss Malvern, the flash consisted of the doctor perceiving the patient's anger, the patient's need both to express and to share the doctor's perception, and the doctor's acceptance of the anger. The flash was induced (or perhaps the doctor made receptive to this kind of interaction) by the doctor's feeling that he needed to reappraise both Miss Malvern's condition and his relationship with her. Before the interview at which the flash occurred the diagnosis had been traditional (asthma, anxiety and depression). The flash, the mutual intuitive apperception or recognition, or awareness of an important understanding shared by both doctor and patient, had thrown light on a focal area of the overall diagnosis with a suddenness and intensity that could not have been achieved by any other means. The doctor became able to base his immediate treatment plan on this focal area with the remarkable result that the wheezing had stopped at the end of the interview.

Obviously the flash itself is not a diagnosis; it is an event that creates a specific climate or atmosphere, which allows further diagnostic and therapeutic work to be carried out with greater rigour and vigour than in ordinary situations, provided the doctor recognizes and makes use of it. It is thus unrelented to hunches, spot diagnoses and interpretations, however correct and hard hitting these may be. A hunch as it occurs in everyday social interactions involves elements of guesswork, luck and hazard, which in our cases were neither present nor required. The doctor at the moment of the flash was observing his feelings in relationship to the patient. He felt the patient's anger with him, he noticed the impact it made on him, and he related the emotive material of this interpersonal interaction to the wider field of the patient's relationship with men in authority. The event might be named *controlled* intuition; it was used professionally and consciously, although arising from unconscious and preconscious sources. The flash was also not identical with a 'spot diagnosis', i.e. the inspired guess of a skilled professional. Spot diagnosis, often used in traditional medicine, is related to pattern recognition and best understood in terms of *Gestalt* psychology. The success of the spot diagnosis will depend on the completeness of the *Gestalt* presented, the doctor's ability to recognize the *Gestalt*, and his knowledge of the *Gestalt* and its meanings. Spot diagnosis always lies within the realm of traditional diagnosis, with all the shortcomings that this implies. The flash in our case was also not an 'interpretation' in the psychoanalytical sense. It was followed by an interpretation: certain anxiety-arousing emotions (her anger with men) were brought into Miss Malvern's consciousness, and the doctor then showed her that there was really no need to be anxious, because men in authority (a) were not really ogres, and (b) could be prodded into sympathy. But the interpretation was a therapeutic act consequent to the flash and did not constitute the flash event as such. The diagnostic importance of the flash thus lies in its establishing a climate of high emotional charge, within which further interactions may take place, or—expressed

G

differently—establishing a *kind* of focal area, specified by an unspoken agreement between doctor and patient.

The flash is, of course, no newly invented technique or tool. It may happen in any medical interaction, whether in general, psychiatric, or other medical practice. We studied a number of ordinary consulting sessions of some of the members of our seminar and found that a flash had occurred in about one third of cases. Needless to say, the flash had not always either been recognized as such by the doctor or been utilized, but the diagnostic awareness of the doctor had transcended in these cases the boundaries of the traditional diagnoses.

THE IMPLICATIONS OF THE INTERRELATIONSHIP DIAGNOSIS

In the realm of diagnosis we seemed to be working on three interconnected levels, and the level and the efficacy of our therapeutic work depended on the particular level of diagnosis:

(1) We sometimes remained on the level of the *traditional diagnosis*. This is an illness-centred diagnosis, in that treatment and prognosis refer to the illness only—not to the sick individual—and are based on statistical evaluations of past experiences. This diagnosis is produced by means of the traditional method of history-taking, based on questionnaire methods, and by examination, in which the patient is seen as the object and the doctor as the uninvolved observer. The extent and the refinements of the traditional diagnosis are limitless: the more the doctor investigates and the greater his investigating skill, the more nosological labels he will be able to attach, though certainly not always to the benefit of the patient.

(2) We often tried to attain the level of the *overall diagnosis*, an assessment somewhat akin to psychodynamic diagnosis. This is patient-centred, but often difficult to delineate and so broad that a *focus* may be needed, which cannot always be determined with certainty and accuracy, especially in general practice. The overall diagnosis involves both doctor and patient, in that the doctor needs to study his own reactions to the patient, because the patient's relationship to the doctor is part of the diagnostic assessment and the observing doctor has to be aware that the object he observes,

his patient, will affect the doctor's responses and observations. The overall diagnosis and its focus may require a great deal of enquiry, be it by questionnaire-type methods, or by lengthy psychodiagnostic interviews. It may result in the formulation of treatment plans by long psychotherapeutic interviews, which in a sense are alien to general practice: neither long psychodiagnostic nor long psychotherapeutic interviews are really representative of the interactions in general practice, at least in Great Britain, which we set out to study.

(3) Our most successful and satisfactory cases seemed to result when the diagnostic climate as established by a flash led to an *interrelationship diagnosis*, meaning that both doctor and patient were intrinsically involved in the diagnostic process and its outcome. The diagnosis arising out of the flash directly relates to the doctor/patient relationship and thence outward to the patient's life experiences. The patient, by arousing certain powerful emotions within the doctor, may be the prime mover of the flash. In any case, the patient establishes the diagnosis and presents it to the doctor. Both doctor and patient then work as partners in the situation created by the flash. The doctor's questions no longer serve to accumulate factual material, but are stimulants of emotive responses.

The diagnosis so achieved is a *kind* of overall diagnosis, but one in which a focal area has been determined spontaneously, by mutual agreement and acceptance, as it were. As we continued our study of the brief interactions of general practice we became increasingly convinced that this interrelationship diagnosis indeed was the basis of the general practitioner's successful treatments and diagnoses. It was not always formulated, not always perceived or felt, and sometimes even disregarded or rejected in favour of other diagnostic levels. But whenever the doctor and the patient felt that the kernel of the patient's disorder had been touched, some kind of interrelationship diagnosis had been made, however vaguely.

This diagnostic feat was never achieved by the inquisitional technique of the questionnaire, by amassing of facts, or even by selecting a focus from the mass of material at our disposal. It was produced by the intuitive process of the flash.

We, and many colleagues to whom we communicated our discovery of the flash element in the medical interaction, were at first very doubtful of its true significance. It seemed to be evanescent, vague and rather unscientific. As, however, we could no longer deny both the reality and the efficacy of the flash it may indeed be necessary to accept the very evanescence or vagueness of the flash as one of its essential features.

The flash is related to such aspects of the doctor/patient relationship as are often termed 'the art of medicine' or 'bedside manner'. They seem equally evanescent and vague, and are often felt to belong to a limbo of ideas to which no scientifically trained doctor could really subscribe, although it is generally accepted that they are of the greatest importance in practice. By studying the diagnostic and therapeutic implications of the flash we have brought these ideas into the realm of scientific study.

The acceptance of the concept of the flash raises numerous problems, e.g. how to recognize a flash, how to use it properly, and how to teach both recognition and usage of the flash to students and doctors, questions that will have to be dealt with in another context than that of diagnostics.

CHAPTER 7

On Predictions

AARON LASK

As no two overall diagnoses can be alike our work does not permit of controlled trials of therapeutic techniques. It is, therefore, necessary for us to demonstrate the validity of our work by as great a precision as possible in diagnosis, therapy, prediction of the results of therapy and in due course in the follow-up the actual findings observed. The thinking is basically similar to that in general medicine: diagnosis, therapy, prognosis and assessment of results. Problems arise from fundamental differences in important details.

First, diagnostic criteria may be skimpy, vague, arguable and requiring justification. Elucidation of diagnostic detail to confirm the diagnosis may well cramp and distort therapy (see Chapter 2).

Second, therapeutic progress in the interview will modify or enlarge the diagnosis, requiring in turn an alteration of the therapeutic aim (See Michael Balint's comment on 'moving into the patient's position, withdrawing, pondering, moving again into the patient's position and so on'.)

Third, a realistic appraisal of the possibilities of success in our work is essential. Undue modesty in prediction will guarantee success; on the other hand, exaggerated expectations will guarantee failure. Early in the research, when we paid a great deal of attention to the overall diagnosis, we thought about the 'big bang' as our aim, i.e. an attempt to make a big dent in the overall diagnosis. It became clear that in the context of true general practitioner medicine time really does not permit it. 'Little bangs', i.e. slight but definite improvement in some area of the patient's difficulties seem to be a more suitable aim. This is quite distinct from the process of attempting to modify the patient's life so as to avoid situations in which those difficulties cause him to be ill (See Malan (1963)).

General practitioners, like Monsieur Jourdain in *Le Bourgeois Gentilhomme* who spoke prose without knowing it, always make predictions often without realizing it. How often do we say 'She'll be all right in a day or two', or 'I am going to have plenty of trouble with that patient'? Perhaps the chief difference between a prognosis and a prediction is that in the former the variables are formalized and few, whilst in the latter they are vague, multiple and less controllable. Hence a prediction often takes on the appearance of a hunch or inspired guess.

To try to overcome these difficulties we established precise criteria for the delineation of the patient's problems as we saw them, both in the life situation and the interview situation. This applied also to the proposed remedy and the method of assessment of the outcome (this has been described by Dr H. Bacal in Chapter 8).

Unavoidably, our terminology has acquired the tang of a private jargon but the particular problems involved require unequivocal meaning. Thus the diagnosis becomes the overall diagnosis. This, as I see it, is an attempted formulation of the patient's life situation— his past and present, his inner and outer worlds, and his interactions with the illness itself—to establish the hypothesis of the problems which bring the patient to the doctor. Therapy becomes the intermediate therapeutic objective, i.e. what we hope to achieve with the patient in the treatment situation. Predictions are based on the assumption of adherence to the proposed therapy (and latterly on the basis of non-adherence to the therapy), and are focused on areas of the treatment situation accessible to the doctor and hence, in due course, quantifiable by the careful judgement of the research group when presented with the follow-up. This comes under four headings:

    (a) Changes in the doctor/patient relationship
    (b) Changes in the patient's symptoms
    (c) Changes in emotional tensions in those people near to and
        significant to the patient and in their relationships with him
    (d) The value of the work done in the treatment situation.

In the following cases I will try to show how the scheme worked in practice and some of the difficulties that were encountered.

Case 1 Mrs Derby—Dr Sage

A married woman aged fifty-six, childless; her husband of about the same age, a highly skilled craftsman who earned a great deal by private work for the very rich. On the doctor's list for about four years. Her aged father of eighty-two, an ex-Welsh miner, had come to spend his last years with her; he was a respiratory cripple due to emphysema and bronchitis. Her contacts with the doctor about four per year, her husband's about one per year and her father's about thirty per year.

Presenting complaint: Tingling in the feet and hands, with faintness.

Traditional diagnosis: Iron deficiency anaemia and neurosis.

Information known previously: A pleasant woman but hampered by a disfiguring squint, with several sisters in the area. She had never 'bothered the doctor' prior to the arrival of her father. She however had devoted herself to looking after her father since his arrival and the doctor had worked hard to discourage her from making her father into a grand invalid. One month prior to the reported interview her father had suffered a mild coronary attack and all the family had mobilized as if for his death. Three months before this report a 'flash' had occurred when she had been talking to the doctor monotonously about the misery of her father's life, getting up each morning to another wretched day of existence. He showed her that she was really talking about herself—she looked startled and tearful and then sadly agreed. She then changed the subject. When he drew her attention to this she talked about the emptiness of her own life. About a fortnight prior to the present report the doctor had visited the home, where he found her in bed suffering from an incapacitating hip complaint which was clearly hysterical in nature. Her family were dramatically gathered around the bedside. He was able in a jocular manner to persuade her away from the hysterical complaint and in a few days it was all over.

81

Summary of the reported interview: She complained of feeling faint whilst doing the shopping. She had carried a shopping basket in each hand. The doctor looked at her but did not examine her there and then. He asked her what had been going on at home and she told him at length. She spoke in a flat, resigned tone, as if reasonably reporting a distressing situation. She reminded him of the death of her mother and two brothers-in-law in a short space of time, and the death one year ago of her eldest sister who had also been his patient. Once more he found himself having to jolly her along and tease her a little about her wanting to nurse father all alone. She smiled a little and said 'No. My youngest sister looks and talks like my mother. I think that's why father likes her so much'. She fell silent and sad. This came right over to the doctor as a flash and he spoke about her having to try so hard to hold her father's affection. She just sat there sadly and then the doctor remembered about her anaemia and arranged for a blood count and gave her a prescription for some iron tablets.

The overall diagnosis here was that of a proud woman, an ugly duckling, who finds her father's invalidism an opportunity to act out the disappointments of her childhood. She searches for the joys of having her father all to herself but is wearing herself out in the process and does not seem to experience the hoped for satisfaction.

Intermediate Therapeutic Objective: To explore with her the possibility of other sources of gratification at this stage in her life.

Predictions:
  (a) In the short term, the doctor/patient relationship will remain good, may even grow stronger; her symptoms will ease up; the life situation will not change.
  (b) Long term predictions. The doctor/patient relationship will depend on his not being too clumsy with her. Symptoms will vary with the doctor/patient relationship and with the life situation. If the doctor/patient relationship stays good symptoms will not be necessary. When her father dies it is likely there will be a relapse. If the doctor has done his job there should be depression rather than psychosomatic symptoms.

Life situation: she is a kind person, and she will find many friends and interests if she can be weaned in this way or after her father's death.

At a follow-up of one week later, presented at the same time, the doctor reported that there was no anaemia as her HB level was fifteen grams. All her symptoms had disappeared and she was bright and cheerful. She explained her giddiness as having being due to the bright sunshine and her going out without her glasses. She was preparing for her cruise a few months later and had been up to London shopping with her sister. Another flash occurred when the doctor saw her as a powerful controlling woman and he said to her 'You usually manage to get things your own way, don't you?' 'Yes doctor, but don't think that things are not good in the family, they are, they're very good, we are a very close family. I don't want to pretend we don't have our quarrels, we do, but we have them and then make up and we're reunited. We are a friendly united family.'

Follow-up one year later: After this report she had attended for a vaccination with her husband prior to their cruise. Again she complained of faintness or giddiness each day at about half-past ten in the morning (a random blood sugar was normal). The doctor reminded her to wear her sunglasses in the sun. Seen the following week she was well and happy again: she was preparing for her holiday. The doctor saw her with her husband. They had both come for the vaccinations and there was a pleasant relaxed relationship.

When seen after the holiday, she spoke bitterly but firmly in a controlled manner about the widowed sister who lived with her daughter below her in the same house. In due course, the father died without any great alarm in the family. When the doctor visited to write out the death certificate, he found her in the house alone, quite calm, relaxed and philosophical. 'He's had a good life, I've done my best for him and there it is'. The doctor has seen her once since that time, but there has been nothing to report since the father's death, that is during the six months throughout last winter.

When the group discussed the rating scores of this case (see Appendix 'B'), the question was raised whether her improvement was due to the death of her father, which removed the cause and the object of jealousy. The doctor had predicted some degree of depression at the death of the father, but this appeared to be absent. Some work had been done with sibling rivalry, and it was decided that this had played some part in the successful outcome. The final score allotted was as follows:

Doctor/patient relationship	+3
Patient's symptoms	+3
Tensions around the patient	+3
Work done in the therapeutic situation	+2

Case 2 Miss Grantham—Dr White

Single, unemployed, aged eighteen, seen for the first time at the initial interview in May 1968.

Presenting complaint: 'I want a certificate, I've got no money'.

Tentative Overall Diagnosis: A very disturbed, depressed, rebellious girl suffering from rejection. She sat there tired, angry and dishevelled, wearing an old jumper and skirt, looking like a little tramp. Her parents had divorced when she was seven, and she had been sent to boarding school. She could not get on with her step-father and later on, when father remarried, she could not get on with her step-mother. She had been expelled from college and after several admissions to various hospitals expelled from hospital too. She was desperate. 'Nobody cares about me' she said, 'they don't give me any treatment'.

'Don't you think you have done enough rebelling?' said the doctor.

At this point the girl began to pay attention to him and there was the beginning of a change in her attitude and their relationship, which in the fullness of time blossomed into a therapeutic success.

Intermediate Therapeutic Objective: 'To see if I can help her try and change her attitude to society at large and perhaps to certain individuals, parents in particular'.

At the first follow-up a fortnight later, she returned looking smarter and this was the beginning of their new relationship.

At the follow-up in June 1969 it emerged that the doctor had made good progress. There was a good relationship in which she rebelled, failed appointments and so on, but was able to talk or write to him with great frankness and honesty. She had begun to take and keep jobs. Her aggression towards the doctor and authority was repeatedly interpreted. In spite of vast social problems the doctor was able to keep her going and help her to face failure and protect her from further failure. It was predicted that if the doctor could maintain his position and stay put, so to speak, he might be able to protect her from enormous social blunders.

At the follow-up in February 1971 good progress was reported. She was now smart and clean, she had been promoted in her office job, which she had kept for over one year. She had made and given up several unsuitable boy-friends. Her mother had invited her to come and live with her; she considered this carefully, discussed it with the doctor but decided to retain her independence. She lived apart from, but on friendly terms with, her mother and step-father. She used Valium occasionally when conditions were very difficult. She changed her family name and when the doctor congratulated her on having got rid of her father, she was delighted and explained that she had written to her father, trying to be more friendly with him, but it was now up to him. Various crises were faced and dealt with realistically, albeit with the help of the doctor. An unwanted pregnancy occurred and was dealt with quite reasonably by her, the doctor and the hospital: a termination was arranged without any undue alarm or excitement.

The patient told the doctor a strange story of a friend whose foreign-born doctor appeared to be attempting to misbehave with her in the surgery, and she asked the doctor's advice about this. The doctor dealt with this on a factual level urging her to pay no heed to it as it was no concern of hers. He himself reassured her he would never behave in that way towards her. The group demurred at this, feeling that the obvious transference connotation should have been interpreted, as there was clearly room for further work with her level of sexual immaturity.

The group scored the patient's improvement as follows:

Doctor/patient relationship   +3

Symptom improvement   +2

Tensions around the patient   +2

Therapeutic work done. This item had not been clearly elucidated at the time of this follow-up, but it is clear from the discussion that had it been so scored the score would have been +2.

In my opinion these two cases satisfy our criteria. The work was done within the context of accepted general practice. Both patients were ill and complaining. Overall diagnoses were established: intermediate therapeutic objectives worked out, by implication even though not wholly explicit, and the follow-up showed results in conformity with the therapeutic effort. A possible criticism is that the stated intermediate therapeutic objectives were too wide in area, and improvement might have occurred spontaneously or with the passage of time. After all, rebellious adolescents do occasionally settle down, and depressed, middle-aged ladies have been known to improve when aged ailing parents die. The following case shows a limited intermediate therapeutic objective in a much more difficult situation where the prediction was explicit and precise.

Case 3 Mr Disley—Dr Green

A man of eighty-five with a wife of seventy. A late second marriage for both; the husband's first wife and daughter have both died. Mr Disley had required seventy-six doctor/patient contacts in nineteen years with increasing frequency lately. Mrs Disley had required twenty-three contacts in twenty years.

The traditional diagnosis included recurrent bronchitis, recurrent eczema, pemphigoid over the last year; on oral steroids; osteoporosis present requiring frequent analgesics. He was housebound and frequently bed-bound. There were panic calls every three months or so, if the doctor did not visit.

Overall Diagnosis: Superficial in the circumstances: a frail sensitive old man who wants to be looked after but feels guilty about it. The background of this, indeed all the circumstances of his marriage, are unknown to the doctor. The wife was cold but concerned for his welfare, very much younger and active in comparison. The doctor thought the dependency problem has been highlighted by a recent letter from her sister saying that she was ill. After discussion in the seminar the overall diagnosis was enlarged to include the following: collusion between the doctor and patient of which the doctor was fully aware: irritation between husband and wife and also a good deal of irritation between doctor and patient.

The intermediate therapeutic objective was to try to get the patient to talk about his aggressive and irritable feelings towards those on whom he was so dependent. It was predicted that this would lead to a 'respectable' amount of hatred, which would really shake both patient and doctor, but if that were possible then the patient would not be so dependent, and certainly he would become much less bed-bound and complaining. If the doctor did not work on these lines, then one might expect only a slight improvement in the patient's physical and emotional state.

Follow-up one year later: Contact has been reduced to about a six-weekly period (instead of three) and no further panic calls. There has been no more complaint of backache and the steroid dose has been reduced from fifteen m.g. to five m.g. of prednisolone. Only one pemphigoid blister has recurred within the twelve month period. There have been minor complaints of bronchitis and trouble with his inguinal hernia. About eight weeks after the initial report the following incident occurred. The doctor was talking to him whilst he was watching a race on the TV. Suddenly he got very angry, thumped his chair and said 'Stop asking these bloody questions'. He turned off the television set and stumped out of the room, bright red. The wife reassured the doctor that it was all right because he occasionally does this but soon settles down. At a visit one week later the doctor discussed the episode with the patient. 'I am on the scrap heap, doctor,' with an irritable gesture.

'Perhaps if I could cure you it would be OK, but what I do seems to be fiddling about and not improving you'.

This was 'on target' because the patient began to talk about his hopelessness at needing people to help him, but not being able to get well. A minor episode of the same sort occurred months later and once more was discussed thoroughly.

Rating: objectively there has been an obvious improvement all round. Cessation of panic ˙attacks, diminution of symptoms of backache, reduction of the dosage of steroids and increased ability of the patient to get around the house. Subjectively, there was a marked diminution of tension between patient, his wife and the doctor. It must be conceded here that the precision of the prediction regarding the necessity of 'opening the abscess' of the patient's hidden aggression and resentment was wholly justifiable.

+2, +2, +2 was scored for all headings.

The capacity to predict with accuracy and precision is a concomitant of understanding in the broad sense the patient and his interactions as reported in the interviews. On one occasion Michael Balint, discussing the report of an unhappily married childless wife, commented:

'She presents symptoms which are the crudest in the world. Not quite, because she could have presented her anus'. At the next follow-up the reporting doctor commented that the patient had attended at the next interview complaining of pruritus ani.

The prediction is the equivalent of the prognosis in organic medicine, where therapy is altered appropriately in the course of the illness: therapeutic blunders = poor prognosis. In the following case the doctor was able to modify his intermediate therapeutic objective and accordingly his predictions as time went by.

Case 4 Mrs Crosby—Dr Black

Aged thirty-two at the time of the report, married about ten years with three children aged eight, six, and ten months. The husband was not on the doctor's list.

Presenting complaint: Severe pain in the neck.

Traditional diagnosis: Torticollis.

She was the eldest daughter of a large family, many of whose members were patients of the doctor's. She was a favourite member of the family with the doctor because he had a good, though rather superficial, relationship with her and she was a regular baby-clinic attender. She was always co-operative and considerate of the doctor's time. There had been severe primary dysmenorrhoea in adolescence and a miscarriage with her first pregnancy. Sexual relationship with her husband was satisfactory. The neck pain first appeared soon after the birth of the third child. It cleared up spontaneously after one week.

At the reported interview the doctor, sensing that there was something different, asked her '*Who* was the real pain in the neck?' The patient looked the doctor straight in the eyes, paused, and then said that she had been wondering whether to bother him with her problems. It emerged that her relationship with her husband was very bad at that time. He had been doing an extra night job since the new baby arrived. However, he had been spending more and more time and money at the pub, instead of coming home in the evenings. She had begun to nag him, losing her temper and letting fly. They would make it up, have enjoyable sex, but things would be as bad as ever the next day. It had come literally to blows: she would throw plates and he would slap her. She commented that she could just not keep her feelings under control. The doctor responded at once that this was most interesting because at first she had said that she had wondered whether to bother him with her problems. It looked as though there were two different people, one controlled and the other one who just could not keep control. She responded by referring to her childhood. As she was the eldest girl her mother had always used her as an extra help in the house and the patient had always felt that she never got her fair share of attention. Even at the present day, though the mother lived close by, she would baby-sit for the other daughters but not for the patient. She had learned to control her anger and not show it off. She commented that she still loved her husband and was afraid of losing him, yet could not help being angry with him; in fact it seemed to make her even more angry. The doctor commented that perhaps she behaved towards him as she would have liked to have behaved towards her mother. At this she smiled, her whole face lit up, and she said 'Yes, perhaps you're right: I know it's my nagging that drives him out'.

A tentative overall diagnosis was made of a women who felt that she had been deprived of mothering and had been keen to be a good mother herself. She tended to make unusually heavy demands on her husband's mothering role, which he had not been able to meet of late, with the result that her old resentment against her mother had been reactivated and had burst through her usual means of keeping it under control, to the detriment of her relationship with her husband.

An intermediate therapeutic objective made for the present visit was to allow her to voice her anger; for the future, to help her understand how she had reacted to feelings of deprivation with regard to mothering, with the doctor accepting the need to pay special attention to the problems of mothering as they developed in the doctor/patient relationship during the therapy. After discussion of the case in the seminar, the doctor decided to enlarge his therapeutic objective to include paying more attention to problems reflecting the wife/husband discord as they emerged in the doctor/patient relationship.

Predictions were made as follows:

In the short term: the doctor/patient relationship will improve in the sense that they will be able to communicate honestly with each other. The patient's condition will improve because she would be able to restrain her nagging and there would be a better atmosphere in the home. Unfortunately, prediction about the neck pain was omitted. Tensions around the patient: slight improvement would occur in the husband's condition; minimal illness amongst the children; and with the mother little or nothing.

In the long term: the doctor/patient relationship would remain good if the doctor continued with his original therapeutic objective, because that would involve a collusion to avoid probably disguised offers of problems concerning her femininity. Thus there would be an avoidance of aggression in the relationship. Probably he would score a +2 under this heading.

Improvement in the patient's condition: there would be a diminution in the mothering role demanded by the wife from her husband. It is doubtful if this would be followed by a mutually satisfactory adult sexual relationship because the patient's problems of femininity would not have been taken up. Thus equivalent symptoms (e.g. insomnia, more of the neck pain, difficulties in the sexual relationship) could be expected to occur. Under this heading the rating could be expected to be about +1.

Tensions around the patient: again probably not more than a +1. Perhaps a more comfortable relationship with the husband and a more troubled relationship with the mother.

If, however, the doctor were able to carry through his changed therapeutic objective of dealing with problems of femininity in the relationship, then one might expect a much improved picture all round: +2 or even +3 for the doctor/patient relationship, +2 for the improvement in the patient's condition, e.g. the husband able to stay at home more, fewer quarrels in the home etc. and no positive complaints, and similarly with tensions around the patient, probably rating at +2.

At the follow-up one year later, the following was reported:

At the first interview one week after the initial report the doctor was unfortunately held up in his work and was not able to see the patient for half an hour after the time of the appointment. She came in, in tears of anger, with the baby. The doctor at once apologized and said 'I'm sorry, I obviously have not been looking after you properly'. She then stopped crying and the interview followed an unexpected course. She commented how necessary it was for her to have everything well organized, otherwise she felt everything would go to pieces. She added, however, that she did want other people to take the initiative but it seemed as though she had always got to do things herself in the end. At the next interview she began to talk about her husband. 'A charming man,' she said, 'with lots of friends, but he changes his jobs fairly often: he isn't really as steady as he should be'. The doctor commented that perhaps she needed a 'charmer' who was also a steady man; this she smilingly accepted and commented that perhaps she was having her husband's treatment for him. At this stage the neck pain had gone. Six weeks later she was seen at an interview concerning the birth pill. She and the children had been ill with 'flu but she had not bothered the doctor. She was seen four months later with a few twinges of neck pain. At this interview she was a little tearful: her husband had gone back to his old firm with a better job but it meant him being out and about much more and consequently not home until late at night. Three weeks later she again complained of neck pain and a deterioration in the relationship with her husband. Her husband had been learning to drive a car for his new job; the relationship was bad and she commented that if she kept on nagging, perhaps her husband would trade her in for a new model. 'I think it's my turn to be looked after now,' she said. 'That's my cue,' said the doctor, 'and what do you think I should do?' The doctor, during the interview, felt the need to be more potent therapeutically. He ordered an x-ray of her cervical spine and prescribed powerful analgesic tablets. She was seen one month later, still angry but not complaining of neck pain. During this interview she reported that a window had been broken accidentally (not in a fight) and her husband had covered it with brown paper instead of replacing the broken glass. The doctor commented that perhaps he was only papering over the cracks rather than getting down to what was worrying her. There was a long pause while she stared fixedly at the doctor. She then expressed irritation about her husband's untidiness, adding that she felt he had let her down in every way but nevertheless, though she still wanted to be looked after, she wanted to be in control too. The baby had not been planned, she added. (At the initial interview she reported that she fell pregnant whilst undergoing investigations concerning her inability to conceive for the third time.) She had now gone out to do a part-time job. The doctor commented that she was working hard during this interview, 'doing all the work' so to speak. The interview ended when the baby, who was toddling around the room, went to sit on the doctor's knee. This the doctor found too difficult to interpret.

She was seen one month later for a routine check up concerning the birth pill. She felt much better, she had lost weight by dieting and felt fine, and had only rare twinges of the pain in the neck. The relationship with her husband was now much better: he had passed his driving test and was doing well in his job. She was seen four months later when she brought her eldest daughter with a respiratory infection. She just said, when asked, that everything at home was now fine.

In the discussion that followed the seminar rated the doctor/patient relationship as +2. Improvement in the patient's condition was also rated as +2. Tensions around the patient was rated as only

+1. Work done towards the intermediate therapeutic objective; at this time this rating had not yet been introduced.

The patient was seen about five weeks later, complaining of excessive break-through bleeding with the birth control pill. She had decided to stop the pill and practice coitus interruptus. Her intentions here were complicated. She explained that her husband had been nagging her and reproaching her that she was being too bitchy. He felt that this was somehow connected with the pill and did not wish her to continue with it. She said that she wished to show that her bitchiness was not due to the pill but to her own innate difficulties: therefore she wished to stop the pill so that he would see for himself that it made no difference to her. She also felt that by practising coitus interruptus she would in a very significant way be relinquishing control to him and thereby giving him that much greater degree of responsibility in their relationship. The doctor's impression was that this was spoken with sincerity. It was considered possible that this was a disguised expression of her wish to have another baby.

She attended five months later to say goodbye as they were now moving out of the district to a home about twelve miles away. She said that she was sorry to be losing the doctor and in some ways sad to be leaving the district. She added that she no longer shouted like a 'fish-wife' when upset but stopped and thought before taking any action. She blamed herself for having been bitchy to her husband in the past.

After the patient had moved away her mother attended the doctor on a few occasions. The doctor said that he tried hard to elicit significant features in her attendances and in their relationship but could make nothing of it. In due course the mother said that she had decided to join her own husband's doctor. There has been no further information since.

The last two interviews were reported five months after the patient had left the district. The doctor/patient relationship was rated as +2. Improvement in the patient's condition was rated as +3. Tensions around the patient as +2, and work done towards the intermediate therapeutic objective as +1.

This was a rather puzzling and confused ending to the case. It was felt on the whole that the doctor, rather late in the day, attempted to deal with the patient's problems of femininity rather than those of her dependency needs. We do not know enough about what went on at home really, though it must be said that the indications were that things were reasonably satisfactory. Perhaps the doctor should have been more potent therapeutically by pressing on. Perhaps something else held him back that we cannot at the moment understand. This is the limitation of knowledge which is a condition of the general practitioner interview; not very satisfactory, but it has to be accepted as inevitable in most of the general practitioner's work. He is rarely justified clinically in being as potent as he may wish or could be, or in delving sufficiently deep to satisfy himself as to exactly what is going on.

These reported case histories are fairly typical of the style of clinical work we were able to achieve in the research. We think we have been able to demonstrate a methodology that is scientific; diagnosis, treatment, prognosis or prediction and follow-up form a coherent programme in terms which are meaningful in the context of general practice. This includes the spontaneity of the patient's approach to the doctor, the multiplicity of factors influencing the patient and his illness and the time when he approaches the doctor; also the doctor's unavoidable ignorance of most of the patient's true story, and the pressure of his training and routine to attempt to achieve certainty by intensive enquiry. In addition we must add to this the frank impossibility of acquiring as much information as he would like in the time available. This is the essence of the situation. The pressure of work in general practice as in most branches of clinical medicine is a fact of life which, though to be deplored, has to be accepted as inevitable, at least for the time being.

Instead of deploring the situation we can now begin to see it in a different light. The very limitations of the system may act like a pressure cooker in the sense that the patient's unconscious needs have to be transmitted succinctly whatever the details of the clinical situation. It is in this area of urgency and compression of communication that the flash is located. We should not expect or wait for a lucid verbalized conceptualization from the patient. We have to trust our own feelings here: if they are right it will come out right in the follow-up. When we have predicted accurately often

94

enough, then we can begin to claim validity for our methodology.

It required a great deal of work in research of time, effort and disappointment to reach the sort of understanding concerned with the concept of the flash. This occurred about two-thirds of the way through the research. We are not unduly sanguine in our claims. We consider that we have demonstrated that it is possible on occasions to make a valid overall diagnosis, to establish a therapeutic objective, and to predict the outcome with some accuracy with worthwhile part improvement of part problems of our patients. As the description of the flash technique discloses, we have to accept and tolerate the discomfort of our own ignorance whilst allowing the patient to 'use the doctor'. In this therapeutic situation with the doctor 'attentively relaxed', flash communications may be recognized and then used with the patient. This will be a very restricted area of the patient's problems, but it is the patient's communication and, therefore, intensely meaningful. It short-circuits the long psychotherapeutic assessment (which is not available anyhow) and, if correctly used with the patient, clinical improvement should be predictable and demonstrable in the follow-up.

We should be quite clear as to the nature of this proposition. We do not suggest that this research applies to most of the general practitioner's work. We are concerned with the quite substantial minority who come with emotional difficulties, overt or covert, which far outweigh the content of the traditional diagnosis. We may ignore them, give drugs, refer the patient elsewhere, probe half-heartedly for an obvious lead, practice the technique of *Randwahl* (if a mentally defective child is proffered a choice of objects, it will avoid the problem of choice by taking the nearest object) as a therapeutic focus, or grit our teeth and settle down to as long an interview as we can afford. We claim that in this area of clinical work our technique is valid, economic in time and usage of resources in the National Health Service, and most important of all, logically sound. We may think we know what is best for the patient, but the limiting factor will be what the patient can tolerate. What he *wants* may be an unsuitable basis for therapy, what *we* think he needs may be too far ahead for him. It must be remembered we are discussing the situation in general practice, not in a formal psychiatric interview. By letting the patient 'use the doctor' we at least will learn more of what the patient thinks the trouble is: what Michael Balint called 'The Autogenous Diagnosis'. By 'using the doctor' we do not imply giving in to the patient's wishes, but the doctor's acceptance of a clinical focus in the doctor/patient transaction. The desired optimum result should not be based on the doctor's view of the problem (iatrogenous diagnosis), but on a careful assessment of how far the patient can 'go with him' in the therapy. The nearer we are to the patient in this respect, the better the prospects. Short of a full-scale psychotherapeutic assessment, this may be the best means of getting to the patient's needs. What initially seemed to be an abdication of the doctor's role may now be seen as an example of *reculer pour mieux sauter*.

This psychological spatial metaphor of relationships is not fanciful. We had many examples which demonstrated how, in spite of —or rather because of—the doctor's sincere efforts and beliefs, the patient had to withdraw from him (as occurred in Case 4).

When the doctor moves too far into the patient's position on the other hand, accepting for the sake of therapy the patient's view of the situation, we often find a collusion index where the doctor/patient relationship is far better than the relationship with other significant figures and therapeutic progress is restricted, as occurred in Case 4. This is more fully discussed in the chapter on follow-ups.

CHAPTER 8

Validation of the Research

*A critical look at the structure of the research
and the problems of assessment*

HOWARD A. BACAL

The aim of this research was two-fold:
(1) To study the ways in which a general practitioner could do patient-orientated medicine during a ten to fifteen minute contact with his patient, i.e. in the course of his everyday work.
(2) To assess the effectiveness of the treatments studied.
The first aim comprises the major theme of this book and is discussed in its various aspects in the book. It is the second aim which I shall concentrate on here.
The general introduction of any new treatment ought to be preceded by a careful trial of its effectiveness. This imperative should not have to be stated, but ought to have the ring of a platitude as the result of constant observance. Sadly, this is not the case, and all too many new therapy attempts are turned loose on the public when they have been judged by enthusiasm and little more. Then they are condemned with the same lack of justification—e.g. on the basis of prejudice and individual disappointment. The treatment which is most frequently involved in this process is what we call psychotherapy, in its many forms. It is fair to say that the psychotherapies have rarely had a proper trial or assessment. It is also well recognized that it is not an easy task to carry these out. Although patient-orientated medicine differs from formal psychotherapy in many important ways, the crucial role played in it by the doctor/patient relationship raises problems of assessment which are closer to those posed by psychotherapy than by the treatments where psychotherapeutic procedures are not involved.
The literature is by now replete with critical discussion with

97

regard to content and design for studies in psychotherapy evaluation. I propose to spare the reader and myself the task of a further review of this literature here but, rather, I should like to offer the following four criteria which I consider must be satisfied if a clinical trial of any treatment procedure in patient-orientated medicine is to be adequate.

CRITERIA OF AN ADEQUATE CLINICAL TRIAL IN PATIENT-ORIENTATED MEDICINE

1. The clinical trial must be designed to provide valid answers to the following question:

How well will this particular treatment, in a particular doctor's hands, produce this result (specified) in this patient (specified) who has this illness (specified)?

Few clinical trials involve such high standards with respect to specificity of assessment variables. But the approach to medical care introduced more than fifteen years ago by Michael Balint in his book *The Doctor, His Patient and the Illness* commits us to these standards. For our purposes, a fourth variable, always there, must be explicitly stated: 'His treatment'. Thus our trial must include a careful assessment of the interaction of these four factors: the doctor, his treatment, his patient and the illness.

2. To be adequate, a clinical trial must be designed so that its results are evaluated on the basis of assessment criteria which have already passed a reasonable test of reliability.

3. The data upon which the results are judged must be clearly evident, to permit evaluation by other workers.

4. Finally, a clinical trial must be carried out in a setting and under conditions comparable to those which obtain where the treatment will eventually be employed.

I propose to discuss our research, in this chapter, in terms of these four criteria.

1. As the aim of the research was to study the ways in which a general practitioner could do effective patient-orientated medicine during a ten to fifteen minute contact with his patient, each of the eight GP members of the seminar was asked to present cases in which

he felt he had done this. Our method of considering these presentations is reflected in the forms of the initial report and for the follow-up. These forms are discussed at length in Chapter 5. Here I should like to consider what I believe to comprise their procedural essence, and thus the cornerstones, of the group's methodology. On the basis of a critical scrutiny of the *doctor/patient inter-action*, plus facts known about the patient already, e.g. from other GPs, relatives, etc., an *overall diagnosis* (see Chapter 6) was evolved. On the basis of both of these, *decisions for therapy* were formulated. *Predictions* were then made with respect to: the development of the doctor/patient relationship, improvement in the patient's symptoms, and changes in the tensions around the patient (the patient's life-situation). When the follow-up of the patient was reported, the above process was repeated, appropriate revisions were made and recorded, and in addition the 3 predictive categories, referred to above, were rated by the group according to scales devised for the purpose (see Appendix 'B').

Let us take a look once more at the first criterion which I have suggested must be fulfilled if a clinical trial is to be accepted as adequate: that the trial must be designed to provide valid answers to the following question: how well will this treatment, in a particular doctor's hands, produce this particular result in this particular patient who has this particular illness? It can be seen that the procedure described above, if it can be carried out properly, provides a structure in which this question could be answered and thus fulfills this first criterion. However, for some time the attempts to satisfy this condition gave the group recurrent headaches for which, true to the practice of medicine, only limited cures could be found.

In this research there was no control group, in the usual sense. A glance at criterion 1 will show that the use of an ordinary control group methodology would be inadequate. The patient must, so to speak, be his own control, and therefore predictions constitute the sole means of permitting a valid assessment of any therapeutic procedure. However, unless one is careful to make predictions which are close to objectives which are both reasonable and possible, the predictions can easily be unrealistic (too high or too low). We may then fall into the methodological trap of making predictions which are either impossible to fulfil or which are fulfillable regardless of treatment instituted. If predictions are realistic then this method provides a workable, although admittedly not perfect, answer to the perennial criticism levelled at clinical research: that it is impossible to assess the effectiveness of a therapeutic procedure because so many uncontrollable variables are functioning.

The next important question to consider, therefore, is what would constitute a realistic prediction in any particular case? In other words, what is the prediction to be based on? The answer has already been outlined in criterion 1: the interaction of this doctor, his treatment, this patient and his illness. On the basis of the doctor's examination of the patient and the seminar's critical review of it, we can make a prediction about the vicissitudes of the patient and about his illness and, to some extent, even about those of the doctor (for, by now, we know him quite well). But what do we know about the therapy he will use? What can we say about the nature of the therapy, in advance, if we are still groping for, and he is experimenting with, the best therapy to be used? Also, the nature of the 'flash technique' is such that, at this stage of our knowledge and skills, it is not easy to *choose* to employ it if we want to. The group initially seemed to side-step these problems. The terms 'therapeutic decisions', 'therapeutic plans', 'therapeutic aims', 'therapeutic techniques or procedures', and sometimes even 'predictions', became blurred and confused with one another. All of these terms can have similar or different meanings and, in the discussion of a case, it was easy to assume that we all meant the same thing when we used each of them. In effect, the group was dealing with its methodological problems fairly well, but without knowing that it was doing so (much like someone who slurs his pronunciation of a word because he is afraid he cannot articulate it correctly but later learns that the correct pronunciation was essentially there, although slurred over). For some while, however, the result of all this was that there was a confusion of tongues in these areas, and, worse still, this confusion had gone largely unnoticed. It seemed to us, perhaps to me in particular who had the advantage of taking a fresh look at the group (having joined it some four years after it started), that our problems of communication in these areas were caused by the lack of a clear distinction between the work to be

100

accomplished in the therapy situation and the goals outside the therapy situation which would intelligibly follow as a result of accomplishing this work. This kind of haziness, wherein these two areas are not clearly defined, occurs all too commonly in the field of psychotherapy. For example, with Mr Baldock (Dr Green) it was stated, as a therapeutic aim, that this patient 'share more of his failure with his doctor, and that the roots of his unhappiness would need to be explored'. A second glance at this statement reveals that it refers to work-to-be-accomplished in therapy—if you like, a kind of intermediate objective of therapy—not a goal of treatment. One could say, however, that if this work were accomplished in therapy, then we would predict that this man would be able to realize some more of his potential in particular areas (this could be specified in accordance with the details of the case).

Thus we have the following two categories:

(a) Work-to-be-done in the therapy situation.

(b) Aims, or goals, which this work is meant to accomplish outside the therapy situation.

In order to get around the cumbersome phraseology of these two categories, the group agreed to call both of them *therapeutic objectives*, and that the first—the work-to-be-done in therapy— would be termed the *intermediate therapeutic objective* and that the second would be called the *long-term therapeutic objective*.

The main advantages of the schema are:

(1) Process and outcome are distinguished and can be referred to clearly in communication between the research participants (no easy task to accomplish), and

(2) Since process is conceptualized as 'work-to-be-done' (called by us the *intermediate therapeutic objective*) it is not necessary to specify in advance *the way* in which it must be done. The results of this is that the apparent dilemma referred to on page 100 can be resolved. For example, having started the intermediate therapeutic objectives[1] in Mr Baldock's case—the need to 'share more of his failure with his doctor and to explore the roots of his unhappiness' —we can then examine how, and how well, the particular treatment

---

[1] The intermediate therapeutic objective (I.T.O.) became a fourth predictive category (see page 80 and Appendix 'B')

101

approach employed (mini-long, flash, or focal techniques) affects them. That is, this framework allows not only for the possibility of experimenting with and studying properly the effect of a variety of known techniques but also of studying techniques which may be 'discovered' as clinical work progresses. This ought, eventually, to provide useful data for the study of the appropriate techniques to be used for a particular clinical problem.

2. The second criterion of an adequate clinical trial was that it must be designed so that its results are evaluated on the basis of assessment criteria which have passed a reasonable test of reliability. Reliability of assessment criteria is a pre-condition for proper rating. Criteria are judged reliable when the various raters agree on the meaning of the criteria they are employing. The four rating scales we eventually used (see Appendix 'B') were tested by the members of the group several times and underwent three revisions before their contents were clarified, judged to be meaningful, and agreed upon.

The issue of inter-rater reliability, i.e. the question of correlation between the scores of different raters assessing the same material, did not arise in this research setting. All assessments and ratings offered by the individual group members were given and discussed in the group immediately following the case presentation. The score which was finally allotted in each category for each case (see Appendix 'B') was the one which the majority of the research participants held.

However, since this was an 'internal assessment', it must face a familiar criticism: the group rated its own pudding, and it could be argued that what one bakes for many years over a hot stove one finds very difficult to criticize objectively. The instrument which we used to deal with this problem was the enquiring and critical faculty of the small working group, presided over, in our case, by even more searching and critical leaders. If anything, we can be criticized for erring on the side of negative appraisal of our results. Still, it would have been a worthwhile check to have structured the work so that the results could have been assessed also by independent raters who were ignorant of the therapeutic objectives and predictions. This, of course, would have provided the crucial test of inter-rater reliability.

3. The third criterion was that the data upon which the results are judged must be clearly evident, to permit proper evaluation by other workers. Rarely are data published on which assessment is based. We have attempted, in this research, to do this as far as is practicable for a number of our cases so that the reader may assess the material for himself. Selection is inevitable since, clearly, it is not a practical proposition to publish the enormous amount of data collated on our cases. Although all these data could be made available to anyone who wishes to study it in detail, I doubt whether the editors will be inundated with requests for it. As far as I know, no-one has solved this particular problem of clinical research satisfactorily, and we have done no better in this respect than anyone else. We have simply attempted to make our selections as honest and pertinent as possible.

4. The fourth criterion was that a clinical trial must be carried out in a setting and under conditions comparable to those which obtain where the treatment will eventually be employed.

Although this criterion is perhaps less often and less seriously violated than the others, it is all too easy to assume that it is being completely satisfied. In our study, it is true that the setting was apparently ordinary general practice. But what sort of general practice, and what sort of general practitioners? The answer is that neither, in one very important sense, was ordinary: all the doctors participating in the research were highly experienced in the practice of patient-orientated medicine as taught by the Balints, and they regularly carried out its working principles with the majority of their patients. The obvious criticism, with respect to these facts, is that the study was carried out by an unrepresentative sample of doctors. This criticism becomes less weighty, however, when recognition is given to the fact that proper patient-orientated medicine cannot be effected by all doctors anyway. That is, for this kind of work, selection of doctors is probably necessary (Balint, Balint, Gosling, Hildebrand (1966); Bacal (1971)). On the other hand, we were aware that the therapeutic interactions which we were studying had very likely been a part of the 'accidental repertoire' of virtually all doctors whether or not they had had training in a Balint seminar. (The contradiction in the term 'accidental repertoire' is intentional, as this was the quality these interactions often seemed

103

to possess). However, since it was our aim to study the nature and the value of these therapeutic interactions and the ways in which they might deliberately and effectively be performed, it seemed reasonable that we drew upon the skills of doctors who had considerable experience in working with the doctor/patient relationship. Whether, and with what skills, other doctors will be able to put into practice what we now have to offer, is another test which is yet to come.

Another special condition of our research was that the seminar was led by Michael and Enid Balint, whose teaching continued both to inspire and, without doubt, improve the individual doctor's performance. Whether doctors can do whatever this group did under their own steam is, of course, something which remains to be discovered.

CHAPTER 9

Follow-Ups

AARON LASK

A vast amount of clinical material was presented and reported on during the course of research, perhaps 150 cases. About forty-five or so found their way into this publication. What happened to the rest? Were they unsuitable in some way, or were they merely the chaff from which the wheat has been separated?

The area of the research interest was that of the shorter routine general practitioner/patient interview, and the clarification of what had been achieved when the doctor thought that there had been a worthwhile contact. Not surprisingly we were exhilarated with those reports showing good results and downhearted and perhaps uninterested in those whose results were disappointing. However, it is commonplace that there is plenty to be learned from failure and our own standard of failure was from a high level of expectation. The field of research was new in that it was the skeleton in the cupboard of general practice, the 'shameful confession' that the doctor never gives as much time as he would like to his patients, because the time is not there. The techniques used in research were constantly under scrutiny and frequently redefined. The diagnoses themselves required to be reconsidered when the technique, itself new, failed or succeeded. The necessity to allow for the emotional blocks and personality quirks of particular individuals, whether patient or doctor, had constantly to be assessed. In these circumstances it would seem inappropriate to talk of success and failure, were it not for the over-riding consideration in all clinical work – was the patient better or worse for the doctor's intervention? As Michael Balint always emphasized in his work with general practitioners, the doctor was responsible for his own work. What he did with his patients was always his own decision, no matter how often various members would claim that a particular clinical line was taken for the sake of the research.

One of the research instruments was the rating scale (Appendix 'B') which was steadily improved to allow the seminar members to assess objectively and independently, from the material produced by the reporting doctor at the follow-up, the change in the patient's condition. Much time and discussion was devoted to the scoring of the results and, as often as not, the clinical material available led to reconsideration of the rating scale itself. However, detailed scoring in the rating scale was rarely a matter of dispute in the broad view. There were times when intermediate scores would have been preferred to a +1 or a +2, but there were on the whole few wide disparities in the suggested scores. A few major differences occurred when the reporting doctor felt that he had failed to convey the particular flavour of a situation or a relationship, which in itself might have resolved the disagreement.

The 7-point rating scale, as already explained in Chapter 8, is an attempt to quantify values which are notoriously difficult to perceive and identify objectively. One does not try to quantify the warmth of a relationship by the degree of tension in risorial musculature in a welcoming smile, nor the intensity of the distress leading to weeping by the volume of tears. For the purpose of the argument which follows in this chapter, the absolute value of the given number is not to be thought of as an exact mathematical value in the usual sense. It is a shorthand statement of a clinical situation which, if the reader were to question, is readily available in the mass of seminar reports which were produced weekly. The most sceptical can probably accept numbers in the vectorial sense of indicating a trend or tendency in the clinical situation. We though it to be less boring and tedious to offer the reader these numerical symbols when presenting the outcome of work done in well defined areas of the patient's illness. The alternative, surely impossible, would have been the description in extenso of every situation to which reference is made. To reduce further the verbiage, we have risked the introduction of a minimum of coded jargon as follows:

106

D.P.R. = doctor/patient relationship.
I.P.C. = improvement in the patient's condition
T.A.P. = tensions around the patient
W.D.I.T.O. = work done towards the intermediate
therapeutic objective

These are explained more fully in Chapter 8.

In the event, certain patterns found in the rating scales provided remarkably apt summaries of the outcome, lucid evidence of the therapeutic value of various techniques, and an almost diagrammatic representation of different sorts of change in the patient's illness, life situation and relationship. Compare for instance the following patterns (the scores are given in the order D.P.R., I.P.C., T.A.P., W.D.I.T.O.):

Miss Grantham	Dr White	+3, +2, +2, +2.
Miss Ely	Dr Green	+3, −1, 0.
Mr Neath	Dr Sage	0, +3, −1, 0.
Miss Keswick	Dr Gold	0, 0, 0, 0.

Clearly there are very different sorts of stories here. Apart from the intrinsic interest of the fascinatingly different sorts of result, it is useful to recognize this at a glance. I propose now to discuss the various patterns in turn, and matters of interest which arise from them.

Pattern of Success:

Miss Grantham was presented fully in the chapter on Predictions, Case 2. A high score for improvement under every heading is typical of the success pattern.

Mrs Derby, reported as Case 1 in the chapter on Predictions, is of the same sort. The essence of what we felt was a successful case was that improvement had to occur and be seen to occur in the patient's capacity to deal with his illness and his life affairs in a manner considered to be much more healthy, as gauged by the follow-up period. 'Healthy' is the crucial word, of course. Nowadays, it has acquired an almost pejorative meaning. I see it as indicating the patient's capacity to deal with his problems in a more realistic

107

I

and productive manner, coinciding with the loss or great diminution of the symptoms which led him to the doctor originally. Whether the success is permanent is a matter for conjecture and prolonged follow-up. Perhaps further therapeutic interviews may be necessary when life difficulties snowball. No exaggerated claims are made here. What is claimed, however, is that these ill patients were helped to recognize the roots and the nature of their illnesses, sufficiently to adapt themselves to a less pathogenic method of facing their problems. A limited area of the patient's neurosis was dealt with. The chosen area was appropriate because of:

1. The nature of the patient's illness at that time;
2. The doctor's ability to recognize it;
3. The doctor's ability to get it across to the patient in an acceptable way;

and this followed on

4. The joint recognition of the capacity to accept and use the communication by means of a new intensity or switch in the doctor/patient relationship which has been called the 'Flash'.

In Miss Grantham this followed on the doctor's remark, 'don't you think you have done enough rebelling?' In Mrs Derby this followed on the theme of the ugly duckling still searching for her father's love.

Mrs Carlisle (Chapter 4) was the flirtatious woman having trouble with her husband and a vaguely romantic feeling towards one of the men for whom she worked. When offered a long interview by the doctor she temporized and said that she would drop in in two weeks perhaps. At this stage the flash occurred and the doctor commented, 'So it seems I must pay you enough attention but not too much'. She smiled and agreed.

In almost all the cases where success was reported, this sort of flash occurred. It is probable that in the context of the short general practitioner interview a successful outcome to therapy requires the occurrence of a flash.

Pattern of Collusion:

'Collude: to act in secret concert with; to play into one another's hands; to conspire; to play false; to act in play merely' (Shorter O.E.D. 1959).

The dictionary definition neatly castigates the most important element in collusion, i.e. the conspiratorial aspect, together with the implication of 'playing with', i.e. dealing with something possibly serious in an indifferent manner. When the doctor consciously decides to collude with the patient for the latter's benefit, then the picture differs considerably. The collusion then involved is that one or both ignore certain facets of the patient's complaint and life situation, thereby minimizing difficulties that would be likely to emerge in the relationship, the resolution of which would be of little therapeutic benefit to the patient.

Miss Ely—Dr Green

This patient was an elderly, paranoid spinster, herself illegitimate and with a grown-up illegitimate son. The traditional diagnosis included weakness following a stroke, depression, angina, ischaemic toe, and more recently, a fractured femur. She was clearly in the last stages of her life. She was apt to form very warm attachments towards priests, doctors and their associates, but was intensely hostile towards other women. The doctor recognized the intensity of her need to love someone and discussed it with her in terms of her relationship with her 'husband', priest and with her own estranged son. He purposely avoided interpretations based on their own relationship, with the intention of making her last few months more tolerable, and avoiding the embarrassment for her of knowing that the doctor understood her feelings towards him. We may express this by saying that he *consciously* colluded with her need for a warm loving relationship by playing the role of a confidant, an intimate, even a son, never however forgetting his role as a doctor. This was never discussed with her explicitly.

Score: D.P.R. = +3
 I.P.C. = −1
 T.A.P. =   0.

The pattern of the scoring shows a very good doctor/patient relationship indeed, but a poor score for her general condition and also for her relationship with other people. In a sense all the goodness of her life was centred on the doctor/patient relationship, except for a small part focused on the Church; and the badness in her life was concentrated on her relationship with women and with her own body.

We may thus deduce a pattern of collusion where the doctor/ patient relationship score is much higher both in absolute and relative terms to the improvement in the patient's condition and/ or the relationship with other people.

Mr Baldock—Dr Green

This man was an ageing homosexual, largely unsuccessful in his work, in his friendships and in his homosexual proclivities. He had, however, a good relationship with his doctor, with whom he could discuss frankly, up to a point, his problems. There was, for instance, a sort of teasing 'getting on top of the doctor' relationship. On one occasion he presented with an ulcerated throat, a rubella-like rash, and cervical adenitis; serological tests appeared to confirm the diagnosis of mononucleosis. When seen by the doctor, he asked whether it could have been syphilis, and of course the appropriate tests were strongly positive. On another occasion he was agonizingly incapacitated with sciatica and a lumbar disc lesion, eventually requiring hospitalization. He repeatedly denied the possibility of any emotional problems complicating the issue. When eventually he was able to return to work he blandly confirmed the doctor's suspicions, admitting that he *had* to get into hospital to avoid a visitor from abroad, whom he had met years ago in the USA. The latter was a bumptious successful homosexual, he claimed, and he just could not meet him in conditions that would have revealed his social and financial lack of success.

He had many complaints of two sorts. First a 'dirty' group including recurrent boils, athlete's foot, mumps, scabies, skin sepsis and syphilis. A second group of psychosomatic complaints included obesity, dyspepsia, diarrhoea, fissure in ano, recurrent backache and so on.

The reporting doctor commenting on the relationship said 'We have a fairly intimate relationship as it were—we use four letter words—he wants me to be a good chap like him—but never better than he is. My medicines are never quite satisfactory for him. He recovers as quickly as he should, but he says he just could not do without me,' and so on.

After discussion in the group the doctor recognized that he had adopted a role in the relationship that the patient seemed to want. Furthermore, he felt that his 'kid glove' approach in therapy represented his own feelings that the patient was unclean, and this of course was a barrier to therapeutic progress. His intermediate therapeutic objective was to allow the patient to show more of his failure and not need such damaging illnesses.

At the first year follow-up a very good interview was reported in which he revealed shame, guilt and the great distress he felt in his feelings towards his mother. The reporting doctor described his therapeutic technique as permitting undiagnosed collusion when the patient wanted it.

At the second year follow-up it was clear that communication was easier between the patient and doctor. The patient could reveal his feelings of despair as uselessness and helplessness—the 'ageing queen syndrome'. Thus he could ask the doctor to 'stick a bloody great needle into me and inject some strength or something'. This was not used by the doctor as transference material. On a later occasion he was caught and fined for indecent behaviour in a public lavatory. He finally seemed able to accept his position as a no longer attractive 'queen' and to recognize the need to look for different sorts of compensation in life. 'If I can't be young and gay, I'll jolly well be fat and happy'. His 'dirty' complaints have diminished, but the backache and status difficulties continue to be problems.

It is clear that the doctor had made a conscious decision *not* to interpret the patient's communication as expressing the wish for a homosexual relationship with the doctor as a powerful lover. He clearly recognizes the patient's situation. We can say that he identifies with him and knows what he is getting at. But, because of his knowledge of the total situation between them (far more than he can easily convey in the group) he chooses to settle for the lesser but more certain gain, not risking a break in the relationship, and thereby being there, to sustain the patient when the

111

latter's needs become desperate. This is expressed as conscious collusion for a therapeutic purpose.

It must be stated explicitly here that the group did not necessarily agree with the reporting doctor's decision and assessment of the possibilities. Some thought that he might have gained more had he been bolder in his interpretations. However, each doctor carries his own responsibility for his therapy and this must always be the decisive factor.

Score: D.P.R. = +2
        I.P.C. = +1
        T.A.P. = 0.

The outcome of therapy often serves as a test of the degree of unconscious collusion. When the degree of collusion is high, therapy often fails. If therapy succeeds no collusion or minimal collusion is present, rather a sensitive identification with the patient's needs. This Michael Balint has described elsewhere as the capacity to move in with the patient, withdraw, assess, and move in again; so very difficult in the GP patient contact.

However, in this case again a pattern of conscious collusion is evident: the D.P.R. score is much higher absolutely and relatively to the I.P.C. and the T.A.P.

Mr Boston—Dr Black

A married man in his late thirties, with a wife and three children. His wife suffered from depression for many years and had been treated both by the reporting doctor and various hospitals with little success. Several years ago Mr Boston had been involved in a road accident, suffering head injuries and backache for a long period of time. In the present report he attended, complaining of irritability with the children: there was a traditional diagnosis of reactive depression. His attitude towards the doctor was on a 'man to man' basis, appearing to wish to let off steam. The doctor hoped to establish a worthwhile contact with him but the patient 'closed down' in his response, being perhaps less irritable.

A summary of the group's criticism of the reporting doctor's technique was as follows: 'The patient is unable to make his wife

112

happy and she seems unable to give; the marriage itself is neurotic. The husband and the doctor appear to club together to fight this formidable woman, who seems however to have something worthwhile about her. The husband appears beaten, but the guilt he is now exhibiting for the first time may be a hopeful sign.'

A follow-up after four months showed that he had not attended and it appeared that he had withdrawn from the doctor. A follow-up three years later revealed that there had been two episodes of relapse of his condition of low back pain with sciatica. The following question had been raised by Michael Balint:

The question: 'Is this a medical problem? Is this man's way of life the kind of grumbling weakness, putting every blame on his wife, the right sort of life? Should the reporting doctor have tried to change it or should he accept it?'

At the three year follow-up the patient said, whilst complaining of a swollen knee which had occurred after he had done some heavy lifting, 'It is not my usual creeping up lark'. 'What do you mean?' 'Life has been good this last summer, we've been camping every weekend and the family has enjoyed itself. I hurt my knee at the camp'.

Dr Black: 'It appears as if your backache was because you were unhappy before'.

'Yes I think so, but I feel fine now except for yesterday's accident'.

Dr Black: 'It seems as if the summer has come to an end with a bang'.

'Well I've had the family down in the camp for another week and I am looking after myself this week'.

The patient returned one week later to say that his back was better but his knee was worse.

Dr Black: 'What has your wife done this time?'

The patient laughed mirthlessly: 'She was too tired for sex as usual', he said. He then went on to complain of the pain in his arms and chest which had lasted for a brief time. The doctor examined him carefully but found no evidence of heart disease. The patient commented that he felt that he had no recognition from his family. If he stayed on holiday with them he would be accused of being

113

a bad provider, and if he did not stay he would be accused of being an absent husband and father. 'I lose either way.' he said. 'I've got to grit my teeth and get on with it.' Five days later he suffered a severe coronary thrombosis. Cardiac arrest occurred within five minutes of hospital admission. It emerged later on that there had been a quarrel with one of his daughters the previous night. The patient in due course recovered and went for rehabilitation. He visited the doctor again.

'So they are looking after you all right now?'

'You can say that, doc.'

'Is that what you really wanted?'

'How do you mean?'

'When you told me about that "creeping up" lark'.

'Oh I see what you mean—well I wouldn't want that lot over again'.

Score: D.P.R. $= +1$
       I.P.C. $= -1$
       T.A.P. $= -1$.

It is clear that the doctor/patient relationship is scored in absolute and relative terms at a much higher level than that of the patient's condition and tensions around the patient; this suggests a pattern of unconscious collusion.

In the discussion Dr Black responded tartly to the suggestion of collusion: 'This is the old, old collusion business. The doctor can't be right because by being hauled over the coals in the past for not patting this chap on the back and identifying with him as being a poor chap—when I don't do it I'm wrong, when I do it I'm wrong—so you have to decide which is right'.

This comment of the reporting doctor is remarkably similar to that of the patient concerning his status with his family, where he claims that everything he does must be wrong. Is it reasonable to claim that there is at least some unconscious identification with the patient here? Michael Balint, in Chapter I, refers to the inevitable dangers of the high degree of identification demanded by our new techniques. In this case the element of collusion in the doctor's sympathy with the patient is well-nigh blatant.

Mr Thornton—Dr Black

A married man in his fifties with a minor clerical job. One divorced daughter with a baby, leading a loose, immoral life, to the distress of the parents. She was under a psychiatrist, suffering from depression, and had attempted suicide a short time before the present report. The patient's wife aged fifty suffers from depression and post menopausal bleeding, but refuses to attend hospital for investigation.

The patient had attended complaining of diarrhoea on three occasions, and suddenly blurted out his fears and anxieties to the doctor. About five members of his family had died in their fifties.

The group thought that this was a case of a usually self-contained man caught off balance, whether from concern over his daughter or himself it was not yet possible to decide. The doctor allowed him to air his fear of death. Perhaps the doctor was worried about the patient dying of heart disease.

At the follow-up two years later it was reported that the patient had attended several months after the reported interview, complaining of piles and chronic ear disease. On that occasion the doctor explored the patient's anxiety about his siblings' deaths and his fear of heart disease. About one year later the patient attended again, complaining bitterly about his daughter. 'I nearly strangled my daughter last night'. She had left the baby with her mother and had gone out drinking with coloured men. She had come back rolling drunk and the patient could barely contain his anger. His attitude in the interview included a large element of whining in self-justificatory reproach: 'What have I done to deserve a daughter like this? Where have I gone wrong?' and so on. The doctor commented that the relationship with the daughter would be used only when there was a crisis. He felt that the patient was not prepared to work with his feelings with the doctor.

The group thought it to be a clear advance in the relationship that the patient could attend the doctor to complain bitterly and openly. The reporting doctor commented, however, that he was aware that he had avoided exploring with the patient the latter's self reproach about his defects as a parent, and his possible responsibility for his daughter's behaviour.

The doctor/patient relationship here was scored as +2 and, though the patient's condition had improved, it is clear that tensions around the patient (i.e. the daughter) warranted a very low score. Here again the high doctor/patient relationship rating and the low tensions around the patient rating indicate a pattern of unconscious collusion.

At the follow-up one year later there had been interesting developments. Nine months after the previous report, after suffering from a mild attack of influenza, the patient attended complaining of tightness in the chest and breathlessness of recent onset. On examination he had a bradycardia of forty-three and was admitted to hospital immediately. He made a good recovery; there was the question raised of whether to insert a pace-maker but he has just returned to work, apparently doing quite well. The daughter had settled down and remarried. His wife had improved too though still feeling apprehensive about the daughter. The doctor recognized that his relationship with the patient has deteriorated. He felt that it was due to the difficulty he experienced in discussing the patient's anxieties about death since his last illness.

Score: D.P.R. = 0
        I.P.C. = −2
        T.A.P. = +1.

As the scoring pattern confirms, it is obvious that there had been a great change in the new relationship. The low doctor/patient score relative to the high score for tensions around the patient is suggestive of what is later on referred to as the avoidance index.

Mrs Dawlish—Dr Green

A woman of thirty, married, pregnant before a planned marriage, and an ex-member of the WRAC. She was tense, wiry and some-what unfeminine. Her mother in her late sixties was a possessive, domineering woman whose husband had died soon after the birth of her only child. The patient was much concerned that Dr Green should attend to the baby's inoculations himself. Much of the time in her interviews with the doctor was taken up with her discussion of the domineering mother. In reporting the case the doctor commented that he had unconsciously allowed himself to collude with her that *she* was not the patient, and that he was simply a rather distant magical doctor. The group felt that it would be necessary at some time to explore her problems with femininity.

A follow-up was reported eight months later. Things had continued in the same vein until the doctor was paid a visit by the patient's mother. He then recognized the close bonds that existed between mother and daughter and the fundamentally anti-male sentiment within the family. At this late stage he recalled the necessity of exploring Mrs Dawlish's problems of femininity rather than the daughter/mother problem. However, the family were now moving out of the district and little could be done.

There was another follow-up 18 months later. Mrs Dawlish wrote to the doctor about a year later asking if she could come to see him as problems were still abounding. When she attended she again complained bitterly about her mother, and the state of affairs between them seemed no different. She felt that her mother was insanely jealous of her, for possessing a son and a husband, but in fact she had left the baby with her mother whilst she had come on this visit. Furthermore, she had become pregnant again. No breakthrough occurred at this interview. She wrote again to the doctor but did not take up his offer of a further interview, mentioning specifically the difficulty of leaving her child with her mother and coming up to London, without feeling able to explain why she was going to London.

This report aroused much interest in the group. Some felt that the doctor should have insisted on her attending. Dr Green felt tht he would be unable to carry through the requisite therapy with this woman under those conditions. The group felt that the collusive element in the doctor/patient relationship which had focused on the mother as a monster, had on the whole damaged the patient's prospects of successful therapy.

Score: D.P.R. = +2
        I.P.C. =   0
        T.A.P. = −2.

Here again the high doctor/patient relationship score relative to the score for tensions around the patient is typical of the collusive pattern. The good relationship is maintained and sustained by the collusive element, at the cost of satisfactory progress with the patient's real problems.

Avoidance Pattern

This pattern is the obverse of the collusion pattern. A poor score for the doctor/patient relationship is found with a better score for the I.P.C. and/or the T.A.P. Something has gone wrong in the relationship, and patient literally avoids the doctor. At the same time he *appears* to be well; probably a 'retreat into health' is the price he pays to keep away from the doctor. It is not clear why or how he becomes well again, and there are features in the clinical situation which indicate clearly enough that all is not well in the total situation. It is quite different from the more commonplace occurrence of a complete break in the doctor/patient relationship, when the patient chooses another doctor either inside or outside the practice and tries to set up a new relationship. In the avoidance pattern this does not happen. The relationship is maintained, tenuously perhaps, through third parties. There is something there that the patient does not wish to give up, though he does not use it in the meantime.

Mr Neath—Dr Sage

The reporting doctor's interest in this case had just preceded the onset of the research project and for a time he had begun to think of husband and wife as one unit. The husband was a semi-skilled factory worker, described as a big, sloppy Irishman, complaining of backache and sciatica. His wife was described as a handsome (sic) controlling, determined woman whose determination can be illustrated by the following story. At the stage of a twenty-four week pregnancy she was able to compel a Roman Catholic gynae-cologist to terminate her pregnancy, long before the abortion act was law.

On the occasion of the first reported interview the patient, about to return to work after recovering from his sciatica, complained of a 'delicate subject' he wished to discuss with the doctor, i.e.

118

his wife's frigidity. During the interview it emerged that both doctor and patient during the last war had served in the same war area in similar units in the Royal Navy, though they had never actually met. A friendly 'old buddies' relationship emerged which the doctor usually found most distasteful. It was agreed that the patient would ask his wife to attend the doctor with the intention of starting joint interviews.

In the event nothing followed. A few months later the doctor called in one Sunday afternoon to 'see what was happening'. The patient whispered an aside that he had not said anything to his wife. An interesting interview followed in which the wife jovially attacked the medical profession on various matters including her own history.

The intermediate therapeutic objective was to help the patient accept his limitations as a man, not to expect too much, and in general to 'stiffen his backbone'.

The predictions were:
1. If the wife co-operated there would be relief from his backache.
2. If not: either severe backache would continue, or depressive breakdown might occur, or if therapy were successful some sort of adjustment to his position would occur, and his backache would go.

Six months later he complained to the doctor of increased backache. He had now told his wife about complaining to the doctor of her frigidity. His manner was described as 'cringingly seductive.' The doctor repeated his view that the severity of the backache was related to his inability to 'stand up' to his wife. At the next interview he pleaded with the doctor to leave the matter alone as he feared that his wife might leave him. Later on the wife attended with one of the children. After the child had been dealt with and dismissed from the room, she began to discuss the problem of herself and her husband. She insisted that there were quite separate problems of (1) his backache, and (2) his lack of potency and her disinclination for sex. She insisted that he should go for X-ray and examination by the specialist lest his back were to deteriorate and lead to surgery. Further investigations were, of course, negative.

The seminar reacted strongly to the follow-up report. The

119

opinion was expressed that insufficient attention had been paid to the wife's maternal protective attitude towards her husband and the latter's protective attitude towards his wife, to the extent that he did not wish her to be upset.

At the follow-up one year later, the patient had complained of pain in both shoulders (X-ray N.A.D.). His wife had complained fleetingly of backache. A few months later whilst attending the doctor with flu during a current epidemic, she nearly burst into tears reporting that her son had left home and had 'gone hippy'. She shook back her tears, refusing to discuss it any more with the doctor and ran out of the room. A week later she had recovered herself and would say nothing on the subject.

Six months later the patient attended again with severe backache — the story pretty much as before. Friends had introduced him to an ethical but non-orthodox clinic, who required a 'letter from the doctor'. He had taken on a new job with little physical exertion, that required much use of the telephone. Again there was a firm refusal to discuss anything but himself or the family or to see his pain as caused by anything other than his spine. He was given his letter, received treatment at the clinic but gained no benefit from it. He did not attend the doctor again.

The wife attended a few months later, complaining of poor vision. She was a little reconciled to her hippy son who was now doing socially useful work. She attended again one year later, seeking treatment for varicose veins. However she refused the proposed treatment on the grounds that it might interfere with her multitudinous responsibilities towards her family. She was cross with the surgeon who would not accept her own proposed line of treatment.

A few months later the doctor saw the patient cleaning his car one Sunday morning and after some conversation the patient in a grudging, reluctant manner invited him in; his wife was much more welcoming. It emerged that they were both probably drinking too much; the husband sullen and irritable; the wife somewhat defensive. Discussing their daughter's plans he burst out, 'At least there's someone who knows her own mind'.

At the time of writing, fifteen months later, neither the patient nor his wife have attended at the surgery nor have they sent for the doctor, though they are still on his list. It need hardly be stated that the group expressed strong criticism of many features of the doctor's therapy.

Score: D.P.R. $= 0$
I.P.C. $= +3$
T.A.P. $= -1$
W.D.I.T.O. $= 0$.

It is clear that the patient is avoiding the doctor, though almost certainly still needing him. Enormous problems and questions remain for the husband and wife and there is probably an uneasy peace at home. Clearly, there must be great disappointment concerning the doctor's failure to help them. They could change easily enough to another doctor or practice. Everyone involved, however, has invested too much to throw it up. There is some understanding of mutual responses and an uneasy equilibrium. It is likely that they will need the doctor in the future and possibly they do not wish to damage the relationship in the meantime. They may well be keeping him for a really rainy day (see patients Mrs Exton and Mrs Cowes).

Mr Quorn—Dr Sage

This man, a laboratory technician, had lived in the heart of the doctor's practice for fourteen years and was literally a stranger to him. He was married, with a son of fourteen; his wife used to work in a shop but soon after the initial report took up factory work close to her home.

The patient first attended with a request for a certificate to help him alter the conditions of his work. He already had a supporting certificate from his chief. He appeared tense, agitated and most distressed. The doctor, who was intrigued by this unknown man whom he should have known, showed interest and concern in his story. At one stage tears appeared in the patient's eyes when referring to his wife's puerperal psychosis. There were problems now associated with the boy regarding his future career; he could not accept advice from his father. The patient had suffered from insomnia and anxiety symptoms for the last year. The doctor gave small doses of psychotropic drugs and arranged another appointment.

At the follow-up one week later the tension had gone and the opportunity of identifying the patient's problem also had gone.

At the follow-up six months later it emerged that the patient had been suffering from difficulty in travelling in public vehicles and in mixing with people. The doctor thought that the patient's developing attitude towards him revealed unconscious homosexual needs and submissive attitudes towards 'boss' men. A strong transference relationship began to emerge which he 'gently choked off'. He gave advice to the patient's wife about her son's educational and career problems.

At the follow-up one-and-a-half years later the following emerged. The boy had started work and was getting on well in his apprenticeship. However, he developed an illness which was eventually identified as abdominal tuberculosis. He was seen by a colleague of the reporting doctor's, to whom the parents turned for advice and comfort. However, when the boy was admitted to hospital the original patient attended the reporting doctor complaining of rhinitis; he also added that he was arranging for his wife to attend the doctor. At the first visit she burst into tears and said nothing. At her second visit she launched herself into a story, with an obvious effort. She reported an adolescent, long-continued and incestuous sexual relationship with her brother, continuing over several years until the latter joined the navy. She had later married and settled down. At the time of her puerperal breakdown she told her husband and the hospital psychiatrist about the incest. In due course she had recovered and returned from the mental hospital to her husband and baby. Since her son's recent illness she had become frigid and had also recognized, to her horror, developing incestuous feelings towards her son. Therapeutic discussion was on the basis of the incestuous feeling having been rekindled by her fear of losing her son, and her frigidity as a defence against it.

Seen a week later, she was relaxed and calm and made little further reference to it. Six months later she complained of pruritus vulvae, frigidity still and moderate depression. Another six months later, concurrently with her son's restoration to good health, she

122

was much more talkative and at ease. She was no longer depressed; her husband had purchased a double bed, and they were both making a conscious effort to improve the relationship. At this date (June 1969) the case was scored as +3, (as we had not yet developed detailed rating scores).

It is unfortunate that the pressure of time and material in the seminar did not permit a further follow-up. However, about one year after the last report the patient attended to report that his wife had left home. It appeared that the relationship had steadily deteriorated. The patient actually knew from obvious clues where his wife had gone and he sought advice from the doctor how to handle the problem. It was clear from the discussion that followed that his wife was seeking a positive reaction from him, and he soon recognized the need to go himself and bring her home. This manoeuvre was successful. In a latter discussion with the doctor she explained that she had become fed up with his passive and generally negative attitude and thought that she was no longer wanted. Further discussions revealed that she had really been upset by her son's developing interest in girls; and her difficulties were centred around this area of giving him up. In due course she appeared to settle down and her interest turned to the question of rehousing, necessary now as the area was about to be redeveloped. When they moved to a new home about four miles away, they requested permission to stay on the list.

Since the previous report mother and son have been seen at regular, though infrequent, intervals; the patient not at all. No other illnesses have been reported and consultations have been chiefly for the son's regular prescriptions. It is fair now to assess the D.P.R. as 0, the I.P.C. and T.A.P. as positive scores.

It is not surprising that the pattern here is again one of avoidance. It may be true that the patient always was an 'avoider', but it is certainly true that he is avoiding the doctor now.

Mr Esher—Dr Sage

A man of forty-three whose wife became pregnant for the fifth time at the age of thirty-nine. He attended complaining of severe retrosternal pain, and it emerged that his very tough mother had died

123

K

around this time. Both the patient and his wife had been ashamed of the pregnancy, thinking of it as a reflection on their clumsiness. However, they soon had become reconciled to the pregnancy, and the family had jollied them along. During the reported interview the doctor linked up the mother's death, the forthcoming birth and the pain. The interview was pleasant and easy and the patient responded well. He recovered quite quickly, apparently, and did not attend for the follow-up. A year or so later he attended with severe back pain following an accident at work. He recovered after a few weeks and promptly returned to work. He has not attended since. Throughout all the interviews he was friendly, co-operative, rather passive, deadpan and non-committal.

The pregnancy was completed without any difficulty and she was sterilized by arrangement. The family moved two to three miles away but asked to be allowed to stay on the list. There have been difficulties; the eldest daughter became pregnant and speeded up her marriage; the eldest son was sent to an approved school, and so on. The wife attends when necessary, being driven to the surgery by her husband who always stays in the car. Sometimes she may ask for a cough bottle for him but he, himself, has not attended since. It is clear that the patient is keeping well away from the doctor.

Score: D.P.R. $= +1$
I.P.C. $= +2$
T.A.P. $= +1$
W.D.I.T.O. $= 0$.

The low level of the D.P.R. compared with the I.P.C. is typical of the avoidance pattern.

Mrs Pilsdon—Dr Brown

A woman in her late twenties with two children, who had divorced her husband for cruelty. She attended asking for vitamin tablets, as recommended by a chemist to whom she had complained of brittle nails. The doctor initiating a discussion of her emotional problems said that she needed something, but not vitamins. She then began to talk about her unhappy marriage and the brutality

124

of her husband, who might have been homosexual. When asked to return after one week, she chose to attend a fortnight later. She then came dressed more attractively and told the doctor that she had been 'thinking positively'. She mentioned having been to a party since her first attendance and coming closer to a man than ever before. The doctor made no transference interpretation. She cancelled her next appointment during the flu epidemic, and on later occasions saw the reporting doctor's partner when necessary.

About six months after the initial report she had written a most grateful letter of thanks to the reporting doctor, which unfortunately, had been filed away during his holiday. At the follow-up four months later he realized what had happened. The seminar, after an interesting discussion, scored this as follows:

$$D.P.R. = -1$$
$$I.P.C. = +2$$
$$T.A.P. = +2$$

The doctor then wrote to the patient at the suggestion of some members of the seminar, apologizing for not answering her letter and inviting her to attend again. This in due course she did but the outcome of the interview was not satisfactory. She was much more aloof and indifferent to the doctor. The latter commented: 'I feel as if I have really invaded her privacy'. What did emerge from the interview was a denial for any need for the doctor or indeed for men in general.

$$\text{Score:} \quad D.P.R. = 0$$
$$I.P.C. = +2$$
$$T.A.P. = ?$$

Once more an avoidance pattern score and avoidance in real life.

Mr Ilkley—Dr Grey

A neurotic labourer aged twenty-eight, with a wife of nineteen and a baby aged one year. He was a pathetic ninny who attended to complain that this wife had run off with a much more virile rival. He was desperate for her to return, even at the cost of allowing her to continue her sexual misconduct. In fact she did return, and a tangled tale of impotence and promiscuity emerged. Somehow or other things seemed to settle down, with the wife returning home and more or less tolerating her husband. Two years later she became pregnant again. Throughout this time the patient suffered from multiple petty injuries, illnesses and operations. He then ceased to attend the doctor and contact was only restored when the wife attended with her third pregnancy. On the face of it, things seemed to be going remarkably well for the family though the doctor admitted doubts about the paternity of the child. In due course the family moved away.

Score: D.P.R. = +1
        I.P.C. = +3
        T.A.P. = +3

Here again the avoidance pattern score coincided with the reality situation.

Stability Pattern

In a number of cases a pattern of uniform change (or no change) occurred in the scores, often after a determined effort on the doctor's part to improve the patient's condition. In the success pattern, by definition, we expect to see all round improvement in the score. What is interesting is that where improvement has been insufficient to claim 'success', it was possible to observe relative stability between the various parameters of the score.

The implication here is that there may be an inbuilt bias in the patient's way of life towards stability; a sort of conservatism or resistance to change, which is not likely to respond to the easily sought general practitioner contact.

The available evidence is inconclusive. It might well be that such patients, on certain occasions, are willing to use a dynamic interview, or have made 'offers' to the doctor which were unrecognized as such. A few examples of this pattern will be quoted before discussing this matter further.

Miss Houghton—Dr Green

A spinster of seventy who initially complained of grief following the sudden death of a sister one month previously. A series of short interviews followed with the patient going through a fairly severe depression. At the follow-up one year later she was found to be lonely and unhappy, and very much attached to the doctor and his family. Score $+1$, $+1$, $+1$.

Miss Hull—Dr Brown

A nervous schoolgirl with a background of difficulty in coping with tensions concerning the birth of a younger sister and her parents' apparent incompatibility. There had been difficulty with her sexual maturation. She had been a bed wetter and an occasional stammerer. The family, who were post-war immigrants, were very close and intensely religious. She had been happy and well whilst away at boarding school, but her symptoms had reappeared with her return home. At a follow-up two years later she had become depressed again and seemed to be turning to religion as a defence against sexuality. It was thought that there had been collusion with her repressions making her a 'good girl' in parental terms.

Score: $+1$, $+1$, $+1$.

Mrs Newark—Dr Brown

The patient was a big fat Italian diabetic woman married to a weedy placid Scots guardsman. She complained: 'A bomb would drop and he would not notice'. She created confusion everywhere, ignoring her diet instructions, playing off one doctor against the other, and the hospital specialist against the hospital workers and so on. Throughout this time the doctor remained determinedly calm. It was thought possible that she needed a fragmented world to match her own fragmented inner life. The doctor remained in touch with the patient's feelings throughout the relationship, at one stage receiving a gift of tinned fruit stuffs ('Don't think I'm trying to bribe you or anything, doctor').

At the follow-up three years later the doctor reported:

'... she remains very difficult to get hold of; she hasn't come in for anything for herself. She continues not to lose weight'.

Score: $+1$, $+1$, $+1$.

Six Minutes for the Patient

Mrs Cowes—Dr Grey

A cleaner aged fifty-eight whose opening gambit was a hearty 'long time no see'. She was a hard-working woman afraid that she might soon die, like her mother at the same age. The doctor, who did not know her, listened to her freely flowing story, told in salty language, without offering any interpretation. She complained of persistent vomiting and mentioned a brother who had died of carcinoma of the stomach. Her last surviving brother had died soon after, from a sudden coronary attack. At an interview prior to her admission for an abdominal operation she said stoutly, 'Give me a good heart, doctor.' Her condition proved to be innocent and she made a good recovery.

At follow-up three years later there had been seven attendances for relatively trivial conditions, none of which were with the reporting doctor. In the seminar discussion there were some doubts as to whether the patient was positively avoiding the doctor, or had taken casual appointments when available. It seemed incredible to suppose that the patient would not have made sure of seeing the doctor had she particularly wished to do so. One possibility seriously canvassed was that she was, so-to-speak, saving him for a rainy day.

Score: 0, 0, 0.

Mrs Nantwich—Dr Gold

A married shy woman in her fifties with a grown-up daughter. She was not a frequent attender. The initial reported interview was quite intense; she confessed that she had a lover, because her husband was so dull and uninterested in sex. She asked at the time to leave by the back door. At the follow-up three years later it emerged that she had rarely attended since, but on one occasion had complained of a minor cystocoele and dermatitis. Her situation with her husband and lover were unchanged. Nothing further of note occurred between the doctor and patient.

Score: 0, 0, 0.

Miss Keswick — Dr Gold

A schoolgirl of fourteen at the time of the initial interview, who attended complaining of injury to her ankle. She was the adopted daughter of an extremely disturbed mother. The doctor felt that he should try to help the girl to escape from the rigid restricted life imposed upon her by her mother, and offered the girl a further appointment to discuss these matters. She failed to keep the appointment and clearly avoided the doctor afterwards. At the follow-up two years later the doctor reported that he had seen her on very rare occasions. In the waiting room when she had accompanied her mother to the surgery, the girl would smile back to the doctor's greeting, but nothing further. She smiles at the doctor when she passes him in the street, but nothing more. At a recent interview she attended complaining of hoarseness, asking for a cough syrup. Again she made no response to the doctor's endeavour to engage her in conversation.

Score: 0, 0, 0.

Discussion:

The question now arises whether such case reports indicate that a certain number of patients in general practice are particularly resistant to this sort of therapy or whether they have a particular need to be left alone. If this turns out to be the case, then clearly much of our work, though not all, with this type of patient has been wasted. In fact, we might deduce certain features in their case histories which represent contra-indications to therapy and thus save other doctors from 'wasting their time' on such unprofitable ventures. It is, therefore, all the more necessary before reaching such conclusions to examine these case reports rather more carefully, from this point of view. In large measure we can put aside the defence or argument that certain cases are too difficult for general practitioner therapy, because the essence of our work is not cure as such, but understanding and the improvement that stems from this understanding.

The first case reported, Miss Houghton, cannot possibly be 'the wrong sort of case' in our scheme of things; this well recognized situation is the very meat of general practice. It is possible that our judgement here has been too strict, or did the reporting doctor in some way fall short? It must be said straight away that it would be a very bold person who would criticize the therapist here, and few would claim to do better in the circumstances, indeed, or even as well. However, in a very full discussion of the therapy by the group, it was noted that there was an uncomfortable collusion, with the doctor unable to deal effectively with the patient's anger and despair. Certainly there is no absolute contra-indication to general practitioner therapy here, although it is difficult.

Miss Hull: In the very interesting group discussion of this case it was noted that the therapy adopted was neither flash nor focal, but a sort of 'following the patient wherever she wanted', with of course a collusion with the patient's defences. It could reasonably be claimed here that a different technique would have produced a better result.

Mrs Newark: No-one had much therapeutic optimism in this case. In the discussion of the second follow-up, Michael Balint suggested the possibility of recognizing the basic problem beneath all the patient's fussing, and thence the capacity for a really useful intervention.

Mrs Cowes: This case seemed to fade out after a promising start with no satisfactory explanation ever offered. I do not think that Dr Grey will object to my comment that around this time he was caught up in other time-consuming work. It is possible that he unwittingly signalled to her a preoccupation, which she might have interpreted as a lack of interest. There is certainly nothing in the case report to indicate it as unsuitable for general practitioner therapy.

Mrs Nantwich: The case report here warrants the same conclusion as made for Mrs Cowes. The reporting doctor was also preoccupied at this time and possibly put less into his follow-ups than he did into the initial interview.

130

Miss Keswick: This schoolgirl was probably 'frightened off' by the reporting doctor's offer of therapy, which stemmed not from the material of the reported consultation, but from his knowledge of the unhealthy neurotic background at home. His prophylactic zeal outweighed his caution. It is likely that further opportunities will occur as the girl grows older, but it really cannot be said that the case as such is unsuitable for general practitioner therapy.

To summarize: Nearly all the reported cases where 'not much happened' show features which strongly suggest that different approaches by the reporting doctors could have produced much more fruitful results. These comments are made not to chide the doctors of course, but to refute the idea that the cases are unsuitable for short contact general practitioner therapy.

Failure Pattern:

I hope we are able to discuss our failures without masochistic undertones, but with the intention of learning from our mistakes and perhaps helping others to avoid similar errors.

First let us accept and then put on one side all the justifications we have for failures. Very difficult patients, experimental techniques, problems no psychiatrist would undertake, situations and contexts in general practice 'quite unsuitable', especially insufficient time; all these are excellent alibis which we can gratefully accept. What this amounts to is that our analysis of failure should not be too much simplified.

How to identify failure?

A negative score is clearcut. Strangely enough, there were no examples of evenly distributed negative score patterns, as there were of success patterns. Observe the following:

Miss Caistor—Dr Sage $-2, -2, +1, -1.$
Miss Exeter —Dr Sage $-2, 0, +1, 0.$
Miss Eccles —Dr Brown $-1, 0, 0.$
Mrs Salford —Dr Black $+2, -1, +2.$
Mrs Merton —Dr Brown $+2, -1, 0.$

This will be discussed further later on.

Apart from negative scores, a good index of failure was the disappointment experienced either by the reporting doctor or the group, with regard to the outcome.

Mr Thornton—Dr Black   0, −2, +1.

Mr Boston   −Dr Black   +1, −1, −1 (see Collusion Pattern). In both cases the doctor was unable to halt or prevent coronary disease, which certainly in the first case might have been predicted.

Mrs Dawlish—Dr Green +2, 0, − 2, though she had not on a straight reading of the score deteriorated in her health. was felt by the group to be a failure in therapy because of the worsening of her relationship with her mother.

Mr Neath—Dr Sage, 0, +3. −1, 0 (see Avoidance Pattern). This man appeared to have improved dramatically in his general health. There was, however, no disagreement in the group that the case had been anything other than a sad failure in terms of lost therapeutic opportunities and the deterioration in the intra-family relationships.

Let us apply these considerations to a few more cases.

Mr Newport—Dr Gold

A married man of thirty with three children: he was a salesman, married to a fair-skinned West Indian woman. The family were old patients of the reporting doctors'. He had looked after the patient's parents through many illnesses. After a variety of complaints, the patient had complained of urticaria intermittently for two years. At the reported interview he had been sourly aggressive about the lack of a cure: 'nothing helps'. The doctor was irritated by this 'attack', and felt that this was a reflection of the patient's irritability. He discussed this with the patient, who commented that he felt so aggravated by his wife that he could have strangled her. He added that the urticaria was worse round his neck, and on one occasion relieved his feelings by bashing the door off its hinges. At a later interview the patient poured out his bitterness about the wife who nagged him and had become frigid and so on. It had been a relaxed interview, like two cronies chatting and smoking in a pub.

The intermediate therapeutic objective had been to allow the patient to feel able to identify with the doctor. A follow-up three months later found him free of urticaria, but his wife was now suffering from pernicious anaemia and awaiting sterilization (she was a patient of a different practice). The patient was much concerned and worried about whether he himself should be sterilized in place of his wife.

Four months later he attended complaining of anginal pains and whilst awaiting full investigations, sustained a severe myocardial infarction. He was immediately hospitalized and discharged three weeks later. After five days at home he relapsed, was re-admitted to hospital, but died suddenly eight days later.

In this very sad case the doctor felt that he had somehow denied the patient an outlet for his aggression by 'depriving' him of his urticaria.

This was expressed by Dr Howard Bacal in another way as follows: The doctor, by permitting too close an identification in the reported interviews, denied the patient the chance of expressing his aggression in the safer medium of the doctor/patient relationship.

Score: +2, −3, +2, +2.

Miss Eccles—Dr Brown

A schoolgirl of thirteen who suffered from asthma and severe eczema. The family was disturbed: the father, a shady character who had been in jail, the mother a drifter from one doctor to another; there had been several abortions late in pregnancy. The doctor arranged monthly interviews in order to minimize crisis calls.

At a follow-up seven months later it emerged that the mother had insisted on attending with her daughter at each visit. Though the asthma had ceased, the girl had grown fat and depressed. The interviews were taken up with mother complaining about her daughter; the doctor found himself unwillingly siding with the mother. At a second follow-up seventeen months later he reported that after a few further interviews the girl defected and no longer attended. The doctor described the tone of these interviews as 'increased reluctance'. She failed to come, he thought, 'possibly because she could not keep up with the standard I expected of her'.

Score: −1, 0, 0.

Six Minutes for the Patient

Mrs Merton—Dr Brown

An impossibly difficult widow who was so very unreasonable and demanding that no doctor could tolerate her. It was necessary for the Executive Council to allot her every three months to a different doctor in the neighbourhood.

The reporting doctor discovered a common bond in their sense of humour, and was able in time to establish a good relationship and *modus vivendi* with her. For the first time in twenty years she attended regularly at the surgery, brought by a young neighbour who had a car of his own.

'I think you are a wicked woman'.

'How dare you call me a wicked woman?'

'The way you treat doctors is wicked—but I'll give you some tablets to make you a good woman,' he said with a smile. She smiled back and something happened between them. The flash that had occurred between them was the mutual recognition of her ambivalence. It was as if the doctor had said 'there is an absolutely wicked one of you but also a nice one and we will find it'.

At the third follow-up two years after the initial interview, it was reported that the patient had eventually persuaded the doctor to call in a psychiatrist. He had put this off as long as possible, knowing that it was useless. She lapsed completely after the unsuccessful interview and treatment recommended by the psychiatrist, and ended up perhaps worse off (except for the fact that the relationship was maintained); the doctor now had to visit the patient, as at the start.

Score: +2, −1, 0.

A comment by Dr Howard Bacal was that the reporting doctor might have confused the medium in which the flash occurred and the good relationship set up (i.e. the humour) as the essence of the relationship itself. He was then unable to use the hostile part of the ambivalent relationship when it began to emerge from the patient, but responded with a kind of hostility of his own, by acceding to the request for the psychiatrist. The good relationship, however, was not wholly shattered as the patient had remained on the doctor's list for three years.

134

Mrs Salford—Dr Black

A childless machine operator aged fifty-seven, who had been married a second time eleven years previously. She had complained of headaches and the reporting doctor became interested as he realized how little he knew about her as a person, though knowing well her medical history. At later interviews he learnt about her extremely unhappy childhood. In the third interview she came in looking radiant and a completely different woman. 'I realize now that my husband really cares for me'.

At a follow-up two years after the initial interview, she reported a road accident from which she had quickly recovered. She amused the doctor as a *raconteuse* and referred to the fact that she suffered no more headaches. 'I wonder why,' she added: but the doctor made no comment in reply.

A follow-up some months later revealed that she had suffered several attacks of gout and a return of her headaches and giddiness. The doctor seemed unable to re-establish the closeness of the old relationship and felt somewhat discomfited. It is possible that things were going wrong at home, but he had no clues. This led to an interesting discussion in the group on the technical problems of the procedure that should follow successful flash treatment.

Score: +2, +2, −1, +2.

The 'failure' in this case seemed to be chiefly an expression of the uncertainty and disappointment of the doctor and the group. One doctor cynically referred to 'Seminar-centred' medicine.

Mrs Caistor—Dr Sage

She was an immature mother of twenty-four with a boy of five and a husband who ran a gadget shop. They lived in a rather shabby, dirty flat, quite different to the clean suburban home in which she had lived with her parents before her marriage. She attended complaining of a boil, depression and tiredness. She presented as a demure innocent little dolly-bird, quite unlike the mother of a five-year-old. She had attended at least fourteen times in the last two years the colleague of the reporting doctor. Her parents had in this period of time moved away to live by the coast, and the patient had moved into her present flat with her husband and child. She now thought of giving up her full-time job and seeking a part-time job, because of her weariness. At the same time she expressed financial need because she wanted to move out to a more salubrious area.

She also complained of headaches and had it in mind to change her birth control pill (for the fifth time). With some encouragement she also added that her desire to change her job was linked to the fact that she was about to be put in charge of some older women at work, and she could not face the prospect of having to exercise discipline over them. Throughout the interview she was quietly obedient and receptive to the doctor's ideas.

A tentative overall diagnosis was made of an immature girl who was finding the responsibilities of married life, a full-time job, a not very adequate husband and the loss of her parents' support all too much for her. Ambivalent feelings towards mother figures and obedient feelings towards male figures were evident.

An intermediate therapeutic objective was formulated: to help her recognize the areas where passivity and ambivalence impinged on her life, and somehow help her to work with them rather than to avoid situations in which such feelings were provoked.

At the first follow-up nine months later, she had begun to dress in a more mature manner and was able to discuss her anxiety more freely with the doctor and with her husband. She told the doctor that her mother had been suffering from a non-malignant brain tumour which had been slowly growing over the last two years. She also added that ten years prior to her birth a brother aged two had died of malignant disease. She felt guilty about neglecting her child and complained of feeling tired again.

At the second follow-up two years later it was reported that at her next attendance after the first follow-up she told the doctor that she had been able to get a part-time job, which would allow her to return home early and enable her to spend more time with her son. The doctor was disappointed, feeling that she was dodging her problems in this way. Although he said little, his disappointment must have been evident to the patient. She returned to the previous doctor in the practice and was no longer seen by the reporting doctor. There were fifteen attendances in the space of twenty-two months with complaints including diarrhoea, pruritus ani and exhaustion. Her son was well and her husband was making good progress in his gadget shop career.

Score: $-2, -2, +1, -1$.

It seemed that the failure here followed on the doctor attaching insufficient importance to the patient's fears and difficulties, and expecting too much from her in facing her problems. She may well have been frightened off by his ambitions for her.

At the time of writing nine months after the last report, before the doctor had time to report to the seminar, the patient had begun to attend the doctor again, complaining of similar symptoms. Nothing at this point can be added to the patient's progress report.

Miss Exeter—Dr Sage

A girl of twenty-one, a clerk, living with her father, an underground ticket-collector, and her mother, also a clerk. A brother a few years older was living in the USA.

She complained of episodes of a disturbed state of consciousness of the *petit mal* type, describing the attacks quite clearly. Her mother had brought her on the first occasion but left the room at the doctor's request.

She was an immature, pleasant but not sexy girl, who spoke freely with apparent wide-eyed innocence. The only problem was her boy-friend: she could not decide on an engagement as they quarrelled a lot about petty things. She often hit him when they quarrelled by jabbing him or digging him with her elbow (just like her mother does to her father?). At a second interview a week later she reported freedom from attacks. Both doctor and patient waited expectantly for the other to begin: a comfortable silence ensued then the doctor asked about the sexual relationship with her boy-friend. Miss Exeter gulped a little and then took the plunge. She is hesitant, her boy-friend persuades her, she gives in and then enjoys the sexual encounter. Lately she had wanted to stop it, she didn't know why, but she felt badly about it. When asked if she went to confession, she said, 'I tried not to think about it, it's six months since I've been. I'll find a priest who just listens to you; you can find some who don't ask questions'. The doctor laughed and said 'You mean like me?' She laughed happily and said, 'Oh no, you don't ask questions.' When asked to return in a fortnight she became pensive and said, 'No, I'd like to think about when I come again'.

A tentative overall diagnosis was made: an immature girl, beginning to face the reality of the conflict between conscience and sexuality. No intermediate therapeutic objective was set up other than to await the opportunity of further exploration.

At a follow-up eighteen months later the following emerged:

Ten months after the initial report the doctor called at the house one Sunday whilst passing by, as he had not seen the patient since the last report and he wished to prepare a follow-up report. There had been no further attacks but the relationship with her boy-friend was unsatisfactory. She was trying to break it off amicably and had begun to go out with other boys occasionally. Another aspect of her difficulties was that she had been a tomboy when they first met but her boy-friend now wished her to become more sedate and feminine. In fact he complained that she used to clump about the house. The doctor noticed that the girl was sitting unembarrassedly with her hair in curlers.

Her brother had married out in the USA a girl who had been an old family friend at home. The patient remembered her and all the boy friends of her brother who had formed a gang in childhood, of whom she was a junior member. Her brother intended returning home in due course.

No further contact was made and at the time of the follow-up report, eight months later, it was noted that the patient had just attended a colleague of the reporting doctor's complaining of scanty periods, etc.

Scores: $-2, 0, +1, 0$.

The group considered that the failure here stemmed from the doctor not taking up the patient's problems of femininity. In the pattern of the boyfriend's sexual behaviour, the doctor forced her and then let her down by leaving her with her difficulties.

Further developments which have not been reported to the group are as follows. The patient's mother developed a non-malignant ovarian tumour requiring surgery. The patient suffered a return of the original attacks and was referred to hospital. A diag-

138

nosis of *petit mal* was made following E.E.G. The patient is now in anti-epileptic therapy; the attacks are diminished but they still occur occasionally.

What can we make of these case reports of failures? Firstly, the pattern of failure is not clear-cut like the other patterns. In the pattern of success the score was uniformly positive. Where collusion was prominent the doctor/patient relationship was good but the patient's condition itself had often deteriorated. When avoidance was important the doctor/patient relationship collapsed but often the patient's condition appeared to be improved (though this was perhaps a false impression). In some of the stability patterns promising cases relapsed into uniform no-change scores. When the patient's condition was clearly worse, i.e. unequivocal failure, each score had a different pattern of irregularity. This suggests the possibility at least that the cause of failure in each case was different. Not everything had gone wrong with the case, usually something was saved from the wreck, perhaps for the patient at least the experience of a shared relationship which at the same time had promise of better things.

In most of the cases defective technique could be identified as the cause of failure. In the three heart cases—Boston, Thornton and Newport—collusion was a prominent feature; the importance of the collusion was that it blocked for the patient the opportunity to use the doctor/patient relationship to work through some of his dangerous aggression.

Excessive zeal, excessive ambition for the patient, the yearning for a 'big bang' as a therapeutic prize for the doctor, could be seen in Miss Keswick, Mrs Caistor and Miss Exeter.

The opposite perhaps, not wishing to endanger a good past result, was possibly responsible for the failure with Mrs Salford.

An overdose of identification with one of the *dramatis personae* may spoil the case. Miss Eccles' doctor found himself working on the side of the patient's mother, and the girl withdrew from him.

Mrs Caistor's doctor was thought to have acted like a father-in-law in the relationship, and Mr Newport's doctor like an 'old buddy'.

Mr Neath's doctor consciously rejected the role of an 'old pal',

139

instead of interpreting the desired relationship, and got into an awful mess.

All too often the doctor saw or used only one part of the equation in problems of ambivalence: e.g. Mrs Merton. The value of humour was evident in cementing a good relationship, but the doctor had ignored the badness implicit in all the patient's doctor relationships. In Miss Exeter's case the girl's conflict between desire and guilt was blatant, but not used by the doctor.

In the stimulating group discussions which surrounded these cases, endless points and aspects of the problems were discussed, which at the time of the interviews the reporting doctors appeared to have missed. It was in time understood that this was inevitable, and indeed this realization led to our focusing our attention on the 'small gains' possibilities of the general practitioner interview, from which emerged the concept of the flash. However, it was rare for problems of psychopathology or psychodynamics to emerge, which were previously unknown to the doctors. What was clear though was that in the heat of the clinical moment the doctors were sometimes far less sensitive to the finer nuances of the patient's comments and reactions, which in the relaxed discussions of the group were seen as valuable guides to therapy. I think that this is an important issue to emerge from a study of the follow-ups. The arresting mass of clinical observations and situations presented so often promised more than was fulfilled. Yet relatively little of it was in the shape of problems and difficulties previously unknown. We so frequently in practice plunge into the security of a decision, a diagnosis, a clear-cut line of treatment, and a way of seeing the patient's problems that abolishes doubt and uncertainty. This is too easily rationalized as beneficial all round, and our flexibility and open-mindedness is lessened.

It is in this area of reaction that we tend to lose our sensitivity to the patient's communication, and in a sense become immobilized. Once we lose our capacity to move freely into and out of the patient's 'position' we cannot 'be with' the patient in the very important sense of identification and withdrawal. I think all members of the group now accept that this is the most promising area of work in the general practitioner context, where sensitivity can be enhanced by repeated practice and the possibilities of flash work correspondingly increased.

At the start of this research my private doubt was about the inverted pyramid of our work, where an enormous superstructure was to be built on the tiny apex of the material gained in the general practitioner interview. This doubt persisted whilst we struggled through the detective inspector phase of our work. The justification of our research project emerged with the identification of flash work where so much movement with the patient was possible when the right setting was provided.

CHAPTER 10

The Time Factor

PHILIP HOPKINS

The medical student at his teaching hospital grows accustomed to watching consultants in the various out-patient departments spending apparently unlimited time taking the case-history for selected patients on whom they will teach. The student is allowed all the time he requires to learn the art of medical history-taking, and also to examine individual patients, both in the out-patient departments and in the wards.

For the medical student, then, it is all perfectly normal to spend time with each patient in a way that he later is to find exceptional when he comes to experience general practice.

When we started our work within the National Health Service, we felt it was sad that its organization, in concept so magnificent in allowing each and every member of the public to have his own general practitioner, failed by making it necessary for the doctor to have so many patients on his list that, on average, he could allow only a very few minutes for each consultation.

After the National Health Service had been in existence for a few years Paul (1952), in an analysis of the time and numbers involved, showed how in one practice the average time allowed for each patient was seven minutes, and in another only four minutes.

These short consultations may be adequate for the doctor to make the more obvious and traditional diagnoses such as the common skin diseases; or to recognize that a lump in the breast requires referral to a consultant surgeon; or that bleeding from some body orifice might require further investigation at hospital.

Thus, for the patient with what may be a simple acute medical

142

or surgical condition, the National Health Service allows the doctor the time required, in terms of referring such patients to hospitals for specialist investigations and treatment. There are, however, very many more patients consulting their doctors day by day with conditions which do not conveniently fit the traditional textbook diagnoses. These patients tend to return again and again to their doctors with a variety of body symptoms which do not appear to be based on any known disease process.

Certainly the young doctor, fresh from his teaching hospital, is very inadequately equipped to deal with such patients whose illnesses so frequently are associated with disturbances of their emotional state.

So it was that there were a number of doctors who had become dissatisfied with their work, described by many as 'sign-post medicine', meaning that their chief function is to guide patients to the appropriate out-patient clinics at hospitals. For the rest of their patients, and these were the majority, the doctors were frustrated by their sense of inadequate training and inability to understand these patients' demands, so that they were ready to accept the opportunity of attending the Tavistock Clinic for the course of seminars in research and training, offered by Michael Balint in 1950.

In the initial stages discussions centred on the drugs usually prescribed by practitioners. It soon became apparent that by far the most frequently used 'drug' in general practice was the doctor himself. The disquieting revelation that very little was known about the timing and dosage needed for this 'drug' led to a long term of research into the nature of the transaction taking place between the patient and his doctor, and the factors involved in the doctor/patient relationship.

In the book subsequently written by Michael Balint, and based on three and a half years of research, *The Doctor, His Patient, and The Illness* the findings were described in some detail, and in the summary and outlook for the future (pp. 286–7) Balint wrote:

'. . . he (the doctor) must find time for his patient and then "listen" chapters 11, 12, 20, and Appendix 1). This, I am afraid, will perhaps remain a real difficulty even in Utopia.

143

However favourable the Utopian economic and medical system might be, the commodity which is always and everywhere in short supply is general practitioners' time, especially during the winter months.

'Still, just as time has to be found at present for a proper routine clinical examination, however hard-pressed the doctor or the specialist is, the time will have to be found in Utopia for a proper "long interview" whenever the doctor considers it necessary "to start".'

Earlier in the book (p. 108) Balint states that:

'Although the need for a better understanding of psychological problems and more therapeutic skill is keenly felt by many prac-titioners, they are reluctant to accept professional responsibility in this respect. The reason most frequently advanced is that they have too much to do as it is and it is impossible for them to sit down and spend an hour with a single patient at a time, week after week. This argument, impressive as it sounds, is not in fact firmly based . . . it can lead in many cases to a considerable saving of time for the doctor and for his patient'.

Interestingly these quotations are but two out of eleven references to Balint's theme of the need for doctors to find sufficient time for those patients whose illnesses appear to be associated with emotional disturbances. However, it was not until 1966 that a serious study was initiated of what could be done, or was being done, in the brief five to ten minutes which most general practi-tioners are able to give their patients, in adapting their skills to help patients of this kind.

A search of the indices of a large number of text-books of medicine of all sorts, including psychiatry, produced a very small number where there was any reference to time. One of them is by Michael and Enid Balint, 'Psychotherapeutic Techniques in Medicine' (1961). Under the heading of 'Problems of the psychia-tric interview (p. 192) they write:

'. . . problems centred around the *duration of the interview* which, in fact, is part of the plan of the interview. The first problem that belongs to this sub-group is *physical time.* Doctors vary greatly in the amount of time they consider adequate for a proper psychiatric assessment of the average patient: some feel that 30 to 45 minutes are sufficient: others like to budget an hour to an hour and a half: and others prefer to see the patient, if possible, on two occasions for about an hour each time. But whatever the predilections—the time available is always limited and is either pre-determined by the doctor's personality, or varied, within limits, by the doctor's response to the patient's needs'.

It was because of this problem, stated so clearly, that they began to ask the question, 'How does a practising doctor avoid a split in himself; how can he avoid being a general practitioner to some and a competent psychotherapist to others?'

After many further seminars in which a variety of subjects were investigated, it was suggested in an ongoing research seminar that it might be useful to study in some detail the actual content of the usual short general practice consultation, with a view to trying to elucidate the factors involved when it seemed that some particularly useful piece of work had been carried out by the patient and his doctor.

In the seminar which met on 21 June 1966, Michael Balint suggested:

'May I just say a few words about what we are trying to do. In general practice we have the painful experience that the technique we developed for understanding the patient needed too much time. The time needed was usually half an hour to one hour for each interview. This was an immediate foreign body to general practice and could be accommodated in the normal run of general practice with very, very great difficulty.

'It had quite good results but remained always a foreign body, and this seminar was called together in order to study the possibilities to devise some sort of method to use the psychological technique and understanding within the normal five–ten minute period that is available for any patient in general practice. In order to be able to follow the consequences of our technique we had to devise some very strict discipline for reporting, for predicting and for following up the results ...'

This was the beginning of four and a half years of study of the short general practice consultation. Special emphasis was laid on the actual content of the consultation, together with a detailed exploration of the factors involved that might be of value in terms of planning the most advantageous use of the short interview. In this way, more patients could be helped by their general practitioners than had previously been possible.

Since the essential aim of this research was to find out whether anything can be done in these short five to ten minute interviews, the cases selected for discussion were limited to those where it was felt that something worthwhile was achieved within this short time. Random sampling was therefore excluded.

Our exhaustive discussions led to the discovery that on occasions the achievement was based on what appeared to be a sudden awareness developing between the doctor and the patient. Once this had occurred, the problem was how to retain this communication and use it at subsequent interviews, and to assess what interval should elapse before the next interview.

In Balint's words:

'The question is what to do at that point when you've got some-
. where? There is an English proverb that you must strike while the iron is hot. Should one do that? Or should one allow a few weeks cooling off period?'

It may be that the doctor must examine his own feelings, as well as his patients'. Some patients can be helped by repeated short interviews, indeed may be unable to tolerate the long interview, which may be necessary for others.

Since a classical psychiatric interview cannot be telescoped into ten minutes, we came to see that this might not be appropriate in the setting of general practice. So began our search for a new technique.

One of the difficulties was that of the doctor deciding in advance that a particular case should be tidied up in the prescribed ten minutes, so that he could report it at the next meeting. This resulted in the doctor trying fruitlessly to find the right answers in ten minutes, instead of trying to define what were the right questions.

146

It subsequently emerged during further discussions that there were cases where the doctor could, perhaps even should, go further in the ten minutes than simply defining the patient's problem. It was agreed that this was a different sort of case that could be called a 'then and there case', meaning that it must be dealt with at once. Balint pointed out that 'this is the technique we ought to develop and we haven't yet.'

On 13 June 1967 there were still differences, as well as new problems brought to light, as shown in the following extract from that seminar:

BALINT: Wait a moment Dr Grey. Can I show you your changed attitude? First you were only receptive; now you make two or three interventions.

GREY: They aren't new. One was 'Is that a good sign?' Then when she got me concerned about her financial position, I had a fantasy of a wage-earner, a son, and asked about that. She said she had no children. Then I asked about her parents and it came out.

BALINT: But coming back, I think Dr White said it, that although she reacted to your potent interpretation about her not having much pleasure, and she smiled and gave you some information, this was dropped by common consent. Again we ought to ask— is it a good technique or not so good a technique? We don't know, but these are highly important details for the technique we are developing. If a patient in the first few minutes offers us something as intimate and relevant as that, should one respond with encouragement, or should one try to get the general picture? If she had been a psychiatric case, it's quite a different thing, but as you are general practitioners, who have plenty of these patients, is it important for you to hurry?

WHITE: Considering forty years have been wasted already, I would say he couldn't afford to waste more time. The other point I would like to make is that this woman has been there all this time—of course Dr Grey hasn't—but nevertheless he knows so very little about her that he asked about children, when in fact she's only had one child who had died. It's a pity he didn't read the notes beforehand, if that was in them. But this, I think, does

147

show how much one needs to explore patients, if one is going to treat them in this way.

BALINT: Again I am not certain whether you are right or wrong. If you want to read all your notes of all your patients, it means about five to ten minutes before you see any patient. Unless you know all your notes already. But this amount of time is necessary first to put them in order—chronological order which most notes are not in—and then read them through attentively and remember them ... in a minimum of five minutes.

ENID BALINT: What is the aim of this kind of interview? I mean I've got an answer in my mind, which is to enable this woman to say that she's unhappy or whatever; but what else does one want to do? Is there a different kind of aim even in a long term?

BALINT: Now you bring in an absolutely new problem.

ENID BALINT: Yes, but do we want long interviews, lots of history, or do we want it to come out just in bits? She tells you about something she's angry or unhappy about at that moment when she's in the surgery. This is the question I'm always asking.

BALINT: What is the short-term and what is the long-term aim? Do you want to take her on for proper psychotherapy? Should you? Or should we give her some antidepressant instead of the tonic?

ENID BALINT: Or ten minutes once a fortnight?

BALINT: You see the great problems and how important it is that this technique that we are now developing, and studying, should be fairly well established and linked up, both with the predictions on the basis of the overall diagnosis, short-term and long-term, because this should determine our technique.

A month later the discussion continued:

BALINT: May I go a bit further now? The trouble is that all your criteria and standards come from psychotherapy and not from general practice, and this is wrong in principle. What we try to do here—that's my idea at least about it—is to try to develop a technique for psychotherapeutically influencing the patient, which is germane to general practice, not an importation. And the one condition of it is that it should be done in the normal routine, which means five to fifteen minutes of work at any one occasion. The question is: is there any technique? Can we devise a technique that would be helpful to continue to get one more step further, and the next step will be done in two months time, or two weeks, when the patient turns up again.

The idea is that your relationship with the patient goes on for years, and if each time you can do a little, one little step, it can add up to enormous amounts, especially if you can use something which is self catalyzing. This would be the idea, but in order to judge that we can't use the criteria which have been developed for judging the normal psychotherapy which lasts—as Hopkins so often reminds us—half an hour. It's impossible. If we expect that, then you must be slaughtered.

ENID BALINT: But look, isn't there something else here which perhaps we ought to look at? It is the way that we, the group as a whole, Michael and I are principal sinners, judge the cases. If the doctors bring along a bit of work which has been accomplished—one interchange of two sentences or whatever—that's looked at and taken to be the bit of work that's done; well then one might go on about what the doctor doesn't know about the case, what he should find out and ought to know. But it doesn't alter the fact that this bit of work has been done. These two things get rubbed in together, so we get muddled with what the doctor ought to have done, and that he ought at some time or another to find out more about the patient.

The discussion went on as to whether the original aims of the seminar were valid or possible, but fortunately by 14 January 1969 the research was making good progress.

Incidentally so was the group, who had now come to call one another by their first names!

At the seminar on this date it had been agreed that two of the doctors would present all the patients seen during one surgery, with comments as to the number of patients with whom they had thought they had done something worthwhile. It emerged that ten to twenty per cent of patients seen in the surgery session of ordinary length had taken part in a flash of mutual understanding between themselves and the doctor, in Balint's words, '. . . you feel that here the penny dropped between you and the patient'.

149

By 14 October 1969 there was still much discussion about what was the difference in the technique of the long interview, the mini-long, and the short interview, and Balint proposed:

BALINT: ... that we retain "mini-long" strictly for the time and then we invent another description for the change of technique? There will then be two criteria which can then be defined ...

ENID BALINT: If we say five to ten minutes short, ten to twenty minutes mini-long ...

BALINT: No, what I propose is the sum total of time: if the sum total of time is two to three hours that's a short case, if it's more than that then it's mini-long, and if it's six months ...

GREEN: All right, that's fair enough.

BROWN: No, I find that difficult because if you have Dr White seeing a patient for an hour three times it just comes in the under three hours, and I wouldn't call that a mini-long; it's only mini-long in as much as the length of time is mini, not the length of time of each interview ...

BALINT: That's why I proposed the two systems; the length of each interview and the technique used in each interview, or the sum total of time.

ENID BALINT: Let's remember where we started: we started with what we call "long interviews" and you can have a long interview whether you have only one or two; you have a long interview lasting forty-five minutes. Well we want something to distinguish between that and the flash, or whatever it is, up to a quarter of an hour but in the surgery, something between that and the long interview.

BLACK: The real thing is that you can't fit a long interview into an ordinary surgery.

ENID BALINT: Or into an ordinary treatment. You break away and you become a psychiatrist.

SILVER: I think we all have different techniques; I use at least six. May I just mention some of the things I do. When I'm dealing with the college cases I have one session there and I do half an hour each, if I'm pushed I might do twenty minutes, twenty minutes, twenty minutes, but as a whole it's half an hour each ... If you know you are going to do half an hour, you concentrate in that sort of way, you can do a fifty minute interview in half an hour.

In another case I deliberately thought 'I'm not going to do more than ten minutes, or a quarter of an hour'. I couldn't do this in the middle of the surgery, my mind doesn't work like that, so I said 'Come at twenty-to-six' and in quarter of an hour I'd close the interview. The other shorter type of case like I had the other day—it was less than ten minutes and I knew I could handle this woman's problems in ten minutes in the surgery, because it wasn't one of those people that one would have to concentrate so much on them. One can just use any of these times ... And I also do the long one, fifty minutes ones as well, the real long cases.

BALINT: We don't speak about predictions, now, about facts—what you have done. And Dr Green wants to record that this treatment was conducted in short interviews, mini-long interviews or in long interviews. The next thing is the sum total of the time spent on the patient—that's also a short treatment, a mini-long treatment or a long treatment. So this should be very clearly defined.

In spite of this, and after three and a half years of discussions at weekly intervals, there were still differences of opinion, which were constantly repeated in terms of the best ways in which the short interviews can be used. This was frequently associated with discussion about the difference between the so-called 'detective inspector' technique and the 'flash technique' and indeed Michael Balint's last recorded contribution to this seminar was about this problem, when on 8 December 1970 he said:

... the question is not whether a patient tries to communicate but how much the doctor can respond to the communication and here we come back to the flash. This is the difference between the detective technique and the flash technique, that the detective only collects material and understands it. How he responds to it is different, whereas the flash technique, if I'm right, is not only sensing what has happened and understanding, but responding so doctor and patient should feel that their talk is the same language and not at cross purposes. I don't think I

151

wrote it down in my paper, but this certainly has to be added.

I still feel that to attempt to help a human being with a problem in five to ten minutes, albeit at weekly intervals, has great difficulties, and may even seem to the patient only to be touching the fringe of his basic problem. Especially as it would appear that a flash may be mutual understanding between the patient and the doctor as to what some part of the patient's difficulties are about, that points to the way in which the treatment should progress. However, the value of the understanding which can be given to a patient during the ordinary visit to the surgery, or at home, was discussed at some length in 1961, and the work on which this book is based, aimed to clarify and extend the ideas put forward by the Balints at that time. This can be seen as a further contribution to the subject.

In an analysis of forty-one of the cases reported to the seminar, eighteen were agreed to have involved a flash, twenty-three had not. In examining the details, six of the cases were probably not within the accepted definition of a short interview, which at the outset was said to be five to ten minutes, and later ten to fifteen minutes; in these six cases the initial interview lasted fifteen minutes each.

A further twenty-two of the cases were subsequently seen for mini-long (fifteen to twenty minutes) or long (up to forty-five minutes) interviews; again, according to the remit of the study these too should be excluded from the results. However of the eighteen patients where it was thought that a flash occurred, subsequent long or mini-long interviews took place in eleven of them.

In summing up the importance of the time factor in general practice, it is necessary to remember that the original aim of Michael Balint's research-and-training seminars was first to examine the content of the usual short general practice interview and find out what transactions took place within it.

This led to considerable discussion and investigation of the doctor/patient relationship, and ultimately led to the recognition of the need for what was called the 'long interview'.

It was then found to be impossible to allow this sort of time-consuming technique for all patients, and it was accepted that we all tend to select certain patients for this 'special' attention and treatment.

Finally, it was agreed again to examine in more detail the exact nature of the short general practitioner consultation and through this further research, the occurrence of what came to be called the flash was discovered in some cases.

It was hoped that this would enable the patient and his doctor to work more closely together in a more intense way, thus making the best possible use of the short time available.

There still remains in the minds of some of us the thought that at best this is simply a method for discovering, or uncovering, the nature of the patient's real problems (covered by the term overall diagnosis) so that further attention can be given to this, either by repeated short interviews, or as some still think necessary, by what Balint originally described as the long interview.

At the end of six years work on this project, there still remains much to be learned about the way in which the short interview can best be used to produce the flash between patient and doctor, and how to use this therapeutically to the best possible advantage.

CHAPTER 11

One Patient, Two Doctors

M. J. F. COURTENAY

One in seven of the cases studied involved a doctor other than the general practitioner reporting the case, a fact which suggests that both the techniques employed and the results obtained must take the role of the specialists into account.

Indeed, to show how central to the research this enquiry is, it is only necessary to point to the illustrative case in Chapter 1, where Miss Oldham had suffered from an overdose of an oral diuretic prescribed by the specialist to control her glaucoma. During the subsequent treatment there was close collaboration between Dr Green, her general practitioner, and the opthalmic surgeon. Much later, however, Dr Green received a note from the surgeon informing him that the intraocular tension in Miss Oldham's eye had escaped control by medication so that surgery was necessary and had been arranged in the near future. This was undertaken successfully and her sight improved. Dr Green had assumed that Miss Oldham had continued to have the usual periodic checks by the ophthalmic surgeon, but had not made a special effort to enquire about her progress.

Because of this the acceptability of the result of the short interview treatment of her problems was called in question because of the uncertainty whether the increase in intraocular tension was an indication of her general state of tension, or whether it was an independent entity. Putting it another way, was the worsening of the glaucoma a symptom shift or a natural progression of the illness?

The problem in all our two-doctor cases was firstly to discover whether the good results of the brief techniques depended on specialist help or whether they are adequate in themselves; and secondly, to understand the tensions which arose in the short interview which led to the patient being referred.

The ideal model of the relationship between a general practitioner and a specialist might be seen as the former working fully and effectively within the limits of his skills until he sees that the patient needs something more, and at that point making the reference to specialist resources which are likely (on a realistic basis) to offer more help to the patient. This implies that both general practitioner and specialist have their useful roles to fulfil, but it ignores the fact that the patient as a person is still the general practitioner's responsibility even when receiving specialist treatment; and it is this question which the case of Miss Oldham raises. How then can the general practitioner proceed? As an illustration, another case presented by Dr Green has been chosen. When first reported Miss Malvern was forty-one years old and held a good clerical position. She had been on Dr Green's partner's list for two years and all her attendances had been for asthma, for which she had been given A.C.T.H. but with little success. She told Dr Green she was having psychotherapy privately, and said that her psychotic mother had told her as a child how ugly she was and that nobody else would want her. She now felt on the shelf and was anxious to be thought of as physically rather than mentally ill, seeing that her mother and aunts were in and out of mental hospitals. She was wheezy and disgruntled and Dr Green suggested she was angry with him. This produced a smile and the reply that he wasn't doing much for her. She then transferred her anger to her boss, blaming him for a stuffy office. The doctor supported her in seeking to remedy this, but also made a plea for the boss and himself, saying that perhaps they were not such ogres, but needed to be prodded into sympathetic action on her behalf. By the end of the interview she had stopped wheezing, though the doctor did not comment on this.

The psychotherapy had been on the patient's initiative. The therapist turned out to be a woman who had known the patient's family, and the doctor made contact with her after he had finished the surgery. The seminar thought it was significant the patient

155

M

divided herself between two agencies, and it seemed that there was some sense of rivalry between doctor and psychotherapist. The patient took her emotional problems to the latter and the asthma to the former. She came with an ostensibly somatic complaint but yet could not make use of somatic treatment. The significance of the psychotherapist being female seemed to be connected with the patient's memory of her mother's remark to her in childhood, as though that was the only important communication she had ever had with her mother.

The doctor's report on this situation left the seminar in a state of confusion about the therapeutic plan: should the psychotherapy outside the surgery be ignored, or should the psychotherapist be considered in overall charge? It was felt that the joint responsibility should be clarified by Dr Green.

The seminar went on to discuss whether a proper overall diagnosis could be made without understanding more of what was going on in the psychotherapy, and it was eventually decided that there was enough information without this knowledge; but there was the danger that Dr Green's role might be limited to emergency treatment for attacks of asthma precipitated by a crisis in the psychotherapeutic relationship. However, it was not forgotten that Dr Green had managed to reduce that asthma with words alone.

Follow-up revealed that the apparent muddle persisted. The patient was under tension but the doctor was not. Although Miss Malvern was controlling as usual, Dr Green tolerated the restriction of his therapeutic role, agreeing to be passive, though apparently useful to her. What was also unclear was whether the picture the patient built up about herself had been achieved by the psychotherapist over a prolonged period, or whether she was reacting to her psychotic mother. It seemed that Dr Green was right to accept that the patient was being protected from a psychotic breakdown by the psychotherapy, and that disagreement with the therapist would be dangerous; even though this meant that the doctor had to abdicate part of his usual role, that of making a complete diagnosis and prescribing the essential treatment.

In the event, Dr Green chose to ignore the psychotherapist, feeling they had nothing to say to each other, and that there was an adequate doctor/patient relationship in spite of one patient having two therapists. This led to the interesting situation of two treatments proceeding parallel without reference to each other. It seemed that the patient needed both of them. The seminar remained uneasy but only asked again for redefinition of the doctor's therapeutic aims.

At the final follow-up report it was seen that the patient had been helped to discard asthma and bring her troubles to the doctor insead. Once she even came straight from a session with the psychotherapist to discuss her problem about sexuality with the doctor instead, as she had become friendly with a man. It was felt that this was a problem which should perhaps have remained firmly in the psychotherapist's ambit, i.e. that the doctor should have refused to discuss it. Dr Green had indeed raised the possibility that the patient was playing off one therapist against the other, but she denied this. She felt she brought entirely different things to each. At the next meeting she brought a book as a present from the psychotherapist to the doctor, but she had mainly come to say she had been promoted. It seemed that the patient was still trying to separate Dr Green from the psychotherapist because of her attitude to the relationship between her parents in her childhood.

Altogether this case shows how treatment used in brief interviews in the normal general practice setting was able to allow the patient to discard her somatic symptoms and bring to the doctor the kind of emotional problems which used to precipitate those symptoms, in spite of having at the same time a more formal psychotherapy presumably aimed at dealing with the difficult relationship with her mother. On the other hand it seems that the doctor might not have been able to focus on the asthma without the work of the psychotherapist, though this in no way detracts from the success of the therapy.

What does emerge clearly, however, is that the general practitioner had a role *irrespective of any other doctor involved*, and it is this which is the most important finding in those cases where good results were obtained.

A study of referrals by GPs made in seminars at the Tavistock Clinic indicates that the doctor's own psychopathology is often the determining factor leading to referral, while Michael Balint has stressed that disturbance occurs in the doctor at the point where there is congruence, or great similarity, between his own unsolved problems and those of his patient and that this leads to a diminution of the doctor's effectiveness. As Bacal remarks, it is also evident that the doctor is drawn to cases which reflect his own problems.

These findings, therefore, indicate some of the negative factors which may lead to referrals, not based on the independent role of the general practitioner but on distortions due to the doctor's personality.

In passing it is interesting to note that the two most common specialities involved were psychiatry and orthopaedics. Although orthopaedic referrals are extremely common in general practice, in the light of this study the reasons for this may not be as logical as they often seem.

This sort of malfunctioning can be illustrated by a case presented in the seminar by Dr Black. When first presented Mr Tenby was aged sixty-two, and worked as a maintenance man in a small factory. He complained of attacks of difficulty in breathing which had occurred several times during the previous week, and which had alarmed him. He had joined Dr Black's practice about a year previously, when his old doctor had retired. He said he had not wanted to consult his wife's doctor, because she was a woman. He had had an undiagnosed dyspepsia in the more distant past and recently had a prostatectomy. He had also had a recurrent phlebitis which had just finally resolved prior to the onset of the dyspnoeic attacks. The doctor was anxious lest he might have had pulmonary emboli, but this was not confirmed. He had also been sleeping badly, but nothing emerged to explain his symptoms, though he was discontented at work and obviously worried about his health. He was prescribed a mild tranquillizer, and he thanked the doctor profusely on leaving, which seemed to be an inappropriate response.

The seminar diagnosed underlying aggression, which would have to be explored gently. At follow-up it seemed that the patient had stood up more for himself at work and this encouraged the doctor to probe deeper, attempting to gain more information about his life and relationships, and a possible sexual difficulty was touched

158

on. The contact concluded with the patient saying that he didn't think he needed to come again. It seemed that the doctor had probed too hard.

Some time later the patient presented with backache and pain in the legs. The latter was found to be sciatica and not a recurrence of the phlebitis as he had feared. He asked the doctor whether he should retire, as he felt the firm were asking him to do more and more work, as the maintainance staff had been reduced. He was very angry with his employers and was wondering whether he should change his job.

At this juncture the doctor felt anxious, ostensibly on behalf of the patient. He felt that the chances of the man getting another job at his age were remote, and felt the need to support him, encouraging him to stay on at work. After a month off work he returned, only to relapse almost immediately. The intensity of the patient's aggressive feelings were now obvious to the doctor, who was himself somewhat afraid of his own aggressive potential. At this point he referred the patient to an orthopaedic surgeon, rationalizing that this was to buy time to get to terms with the patient's angry feelings.

The seminar saw the situation as the patient trying to retire with backache, while the doctor persisted in trying to stiffen him, and getting an orthopaedic surgeon to back up his opinion. This had placed the doctor in the dangerous situation of becoming an authoritarian figure whom the patient had to fight, so making it even more difficult for the aggressive feelings to be handled. It was thought that a better technique would have been to explore the consequences of retiring, rather than trying to impose solutions. Dr Black pleaded that he had consciously been trying to avoid being too probing as he had been on the previous occasion, but finally accepted that he had attempted to circumvent the problem rather than face it.

The orthopaedic surgeon prescribed, as the seminar had predicted, exercise and a lumbar corset, after which the patient withdrew both from the outpatients department and also from the doctor for a while. It seemed the patient decided to withdraw and turned his anger on himself, so that the next presentation was of a very depressed man, in an almost psychotic state. The previous

159

breakdown in the doctor/patient relationship made it very difficult for the doctor to get in touch with the patient's feelings, but he was able eventually to persuade him to see a psychiatrist voluntarily, though the patient was still so ill when seen in outpatients that admission was advised.

This case was clearly a failure and the initial referral to the orthopaedic surgeon can be seen in retrospect as the turning point. The doctor's inability to handle at this point his own conflict, which reflected something of the patient's problem, led him to retreat from the concept of an overall diagnosis, which was gradually being built up in the previous doctor/patient communication. The result was a damaging breakdown in the communication and increased severity of the illness. This would probably not have occurred if the doctor had continued to work with the patient in exploring the probable consequences of what the patient wanted to do, taking into account his anger directed outwards. In short, if the general practitioner abdicates his independent role, specialist help itself becomes much more difficult to provide effectively.

In conclusion it can be seen that the work which is done in ordinary general practice contact is extremely important in itself, and its quality largely determines how effective the treatment which the patient receives from all sources will be.

Epilogue

ENID BALINT

While writing the final paragraphs of this book I find myself looking back over the years and feeling as Michael Balint and I
invariably did whenever a book was ready for the publishers. Ever
since 1956 when the first of the books of this series, *The Doctor,
His Patient and The Illness* was finished, though pleased we were
dissatisfied with the work and were already planning the next. What
was completed was a description of an ongoing piece of work. If
we had waited to publish until that work was completed would it
ever have been published? Or if published, would it any longer
have been of interest?

It is good to know that although my husband died before this
book was even half written the thinking which he initiated did not
stop when he died; on the contrary. Not only, as we said in our
Foreword, did Michael Balint continue to throw out new ideas and
continue in a spirit of sceptical scrutiny until he died, but the group
of doctors with whom we worked, most of whom have contributed
one or more chapters to this book and all of whom have made
valuable contributions to the thinking in it, has continued in this
spirit. New ideas and a critical approach to them have not stopped.
The group gained, if anything, added impetus because we were
all aware that our work must go on and that we must not finalize
the research which was started in the early 1950's.

True, we are aware that the book is not an entirely satisfactory
account of our ideas and that many things might have been said
better and that there are many gaps. However we are ready to

161

publish. As has already been said, the work on which this book was based started in January 1966 when the two of us, Michael Balint and I, invited a group of doctors, who had worked with us before and thus were well trained in the study of the possible therapeutic uses of the doctor/patient relationship, to join us again.

Our idea was to investigate with them what use their training had been to them in the normal routine of their practices. We did not wish to study on this occasion, as we had before, the relationship they had with their patients when they gave them long interviews.

In his chapter Michael Balint said that we set out to find whether new techniques could be designed which would enable the doctor to offer psychological help to any of his patients without disrupting the normal routine of his practice. My own personal interest was more to see if such techniques already existed and if so to see if we could isolate and describe them.

In the various chapters in the book it will be seen that each author saw our task in a slightly different light. In my view this is an advantage rather than the reverse. I think our different emphases and interests together make up the whole, and the book would be the poorer if we tried to iron out our differences. We decided as well, as will be clear to the reader, that each member of the group who wished to write a chapter should be allowed to write about that aspect of our work which interested him most and that the editors should interfere as little as possible with his style and presentation. His style of working and his way of thinking could not, in our view, be separated any more in the book than they could or should be in his work with patients, or in the seminar itself. These separate contributions together give a true picture of our work and show in what ways the doctor can and does help his patients with their psychological problems in the routine of his practice.

In his summary (Chapter 21) to *The Doctor, His Patient and The Illness* Michael Balint said that his description of the general practitioner and the psychiatrist was rather idealized and Utopian, but that it was possible to find general practitioners who were interested enough to acquire the necessary skills to work with their patients' emotional problems; however, for the time being, he said, these general practitioners were rare birds. Unfortunately this is still true.

In the study described in this book, however, a handful of doctors has tried to tackle the problem of whether the skills they had already developed to help their patients in long interviews had enabled them to develop new ones to help their patients during the ordinary surgery hours. I hope it is clear that we are not offering second-rate medicine because of lack of time.

In our opinion our patients will not suffer from our change of interest from the long interviews to our present interest in what happens in the normal routine of general practice. Our hope is that by trying to isolate what can happen during the short interviews in the surgery we have made some advance in approaching many problems, among them those connected with the dangers of a too dependent doctor/patient relationship.

I do not know whether the reader will be of the opinion that we have discovered a new technique. In the seminar there is still much discussion about whether the 'flash' should be described as a technique or not. In any case we are of the opinion that the work and the thinking that this expression has thrown up has been fruitful to us and should enable us to go further in our study of the brief interview in the general practitioner setting. Many of us still wish we could have found a better way of describing this particular therapeutic transaction, but once the word flash was used we could not discard it although we often tried to do so.

It will be clear to the reader how difficult we have found it to describe our work and how continuously the question of the effectiveness of our work has been raised. We are particularly indebted to Dr Howard Bacal who, joining us rather late, helped us clarify our ideas and describe them more adequately.

Finally, what are the many important questions still left unanswered? Perhaps two of the main ones concern how to diagnose those patients for whom a brief encounter—a flash—is the optimum treatment at the particular moment in his life which we are studying; and how to recognize those patients for whom long interviews are the treatment of choice. Secondly, how to train doctors in the skills which we have been describing. I must emphasize that brief interviews of this kind have been studied in the setting of general practice only when an ongoing relationship between the doctor and his patient is customary so that although the flash itself is brief the relationship in which it occurs is long.

The Forms used in the Research

M. J. F. COURTENAY

Enid Balint's Seminar, Card for Initial Report

CASE NO.   PATIENT'S NAME   DOCTOR (REPORTING)

1. Date reported to Seminar:
2. Date seen by doctor:
3. Apparent reason for coming:
4. Examinations:
   (a) Done previously
   (b) At this interview:
5. Traditional Diagnosis as made by presenting doctor:
6. Information leading to Overall Diagnosis:
   (a) Already known:
   (b) From this interview:
   (c) From Seminar discussion:
7. Overall Diagnosis:
8. Prognosis in terms of the Traditional Diagnosis:
9. Prognosis in terms of the Overall Diagnosis:

Six Minutes for the Patient

MARK I   *April 1966*

A. *Patient's Name*   *Date of Birth*   *Occupation*

....

   Spouse's Name   *Date of Birth*   *Occupation*

....

   Children's Names   *Dates of Birth*

....
....
....

B. 1. Presenting Complaint   ....
   2. Traditional Diagnosis   ....

C. Overall Diagnosis:
   Iatrogenous   ....
   Autogenous   ....

D. Apparent Reasons for Coming:
   Iatrogenous   ....
   Autogenous   ....

E. Therapeutic decisions:
   1. Focal Area   ....
   2. (a) Points for   ....
      (b) Points against ....
   3. (a) Decisions for this visit   ....
      (b) Long term plans ....

F. Predictions:
   Short-term   ....
   Long-term   ....

166

FORM FOR INITIAL REPORT

MARK IX   *January 1970*

A. 1. Reporting Doctor
   2. Patient's name   Date of birth (age)   Occupation
   3. Date of marriage (number of years)
   4. Spouse's name   Date of birth (age)   Occupation
   5. Children's names   Dates of birth (ages)   Occupations
   6. Date and length of interview
   7. Length of time on Doctor's list
   8. Approximate number of contacts with Doctor (whole family)

B. 1. Presenting Complaint
   2. Traditional Diagnosis

C. 1. Information known previously to interview leading to Overall Diagnosis, *with special attention to D/P relationship*
   2. Summary of the interview, *with special attention to the D/P relationship*
   3. Research check-list:
     (a) The 'Flash' that occurred in the interview
     (b) Dynamic summary of the interview
     (c) The patient's reactions as observed during the interview to any therapeutic attempt
     (d) What patient tried to convey to the doctor
     (e) What the patient was trying to get from the doctor
     (f) Extent of collusion between doctor and patient

D. 1. Overall Diagnosis
   2. Therapeutic decisions based on
     (a) Traditional Diagnosis
     (b) Overall Diagnosis
       (i) For the interview
       (ii) For the future

E. Predictions:
   (a) Short-term (in terms of D/P relationship, patient's life situation and symptomatology)
  (b) Long-term (in terms of D/P relationship, patient's life situation and symptomatology)

F. Doctor's Afterthoughts

G. Changes and additions made during Seminar discussion

Six Minutes for the Patient

F.U. Form

Follow-up Card of Enid Balint's Seminar

(1) Factual Material

    (a) Name of Doctor
    (b) Name of Patient
    (c) Date of original report
    (d) Date of F.U. reports

(2) Material relating to
    Traditional Diagnosis

    (a) Date and reasons for return
        visit
    (b) Examinations done since last
        visit
    (c) Any changes, additions or
        ommissions to Traditional
        Diagnosis

(3) New information leading to
    the Overall Diagnosis

    (a) From reporting doctor
    (b) Emerging from seminar dis-
        cussion

(4) Changes in Overall Diagnosis

(5) Changes in Prognosis

The F.U. Form

MARK III   FOLLOW-UP FORM   *November 1966*

A. 1. Reporting Doctor
   2. Patient's name and number of original report
   3. Numbers and dates of previous follow-up reports
   4. Date of interview(s)
   5. Length of interview(s)

B. New or changed traditional diagnosis, if any

C. How far prediction of (date) proved correct:
   (a) Short-term
   (b) Long-term

D. 1. New material pertaining to Overall Diagnosis
   2. Changes in Overall Diagnosis
      (a) Iatrogenous
      (b) Autogenous

E. Changes in Predictions (in terms of doctor/patient relationship, patient's life situation and symptomatology)

F. Changes and additions made during the Seminar discussion

G. Discussion of doctor's technique

Six Minutes for the Patient

The F.U. Form

MARK XI   FOLLOW-UP FORM   *July 1970*

A. 1. Reporting doctor
   2. Name of patient, number of original report, and present age.
   3. Number of contacts since last report (average per year—any change)
   4. Number of contacts with rest of family since last report (average per year—any change)
   5. Time taken for original and subsequent interviews.

B. 1. Dr Lask's round-up of the case
   2. Dr Gill's previous summary of the doctor's technique
   3. Previous Overall Diagnosis
   4. Previous Predictions (a) Short-term (with reference to D/P relationship, patient's
                            (b) Long-term life situation and symptomatology)

C. 1. History of contacts and development of case by reporting doctor.
   2. Check list: (a) How far were the predictions fulfilled?
                      (i) short-term
                      (ii) long-term
                  (b) Changes in the Overall Diagnosis, *with particular reference to the D/P relationship*
                  (c) Changes in the doctor's technique
                  (d) How closely were the (future) therapeutic decisions based on the Overall Diagnosis adhered to?

D. 1. New Overall Diagnosis (if any)
   2. New therapeutic decisions based on Overall Diagnosis

E. New predictions (a) short-term
                    (b) long-term

F. ratings: (1) Doctor/patient relationship
            (2) Symptom-improvement in case
            (3) Tensions round patient

G. Changes and additions made during Seminar discussion.

170

APPENDIX B

The Rating Scale

HOWARD A. BACAL

RATING OF THE PATIENT'S SYMPTOMS

N.B. In this scale, the currently known state of the patient's symptomatology is rated. The base-line for comparison is the state of the patient's symptomatology when last reported on.

+3 Asymptomatic

+2 Almost asymptomatic; no new symptoms.

+1 Some symptoms persist and/or some new symptoms of equal severity to the original symptoms produced.

 0 No change in symptomatology.

−1 Symptoms slightly worse and/or new symptoms of slightly greater severity than those last reported on.

−2 Symptoms considerably worse and/or new symptoms of considerably greater severity than those last reported on.

−3 Symptoms seriously worse and/or new symptoms of seriously greater severity than those last reported on.

171

N

RATING OF DOCTOR/PATIENT RELATIONSHIP

+3   The behaviour of doctor and patient shows that they have a relationship in which they are able to communicate freely and sincerely with one another.

+2   The behaviour of doctor and patient shows that they have a relationship in which they are able to communicate freely and sincerely. (Minimal restriction and minimal degree of dishonesty are implied.)

+1   The behaviour of doctor and patient shows that they make some attempt, with some success, to establish a relationship in which they can communicate freely and sincerely. (Moderate restriction and moderate degrees of dishonesty are implied.)

  0   The behaviour of doctor and/or patient shows that they are barely able to establish a relationship in which they can communicate with any degree of freedom or sincerity. (Marked restriction and dishonesty are implied, but attempts may still be made to correct this.)

−1   The behaviour of doctor and/or patient shows that either or both do not attempt to establish a relationship in which they can communicate freely and honestly. (Marked restriction and dishonesty are implied as in 0, the difference being the absence of any attempt to change this situation.)

−2   The behaviour of doctor and/or patient shows that efforts are being made by either or both to avoid honest communication with each other.
(This must be distinguished from the situation where a patient drops out of contact unexpectedly but where the available evidence indicates that the patient is able to communicate honestly with his doctor if the need arises, i.e a score of from +1 upwards. Where these two situations cannot be distinguished, this ought to be stated, and a rating ought not to be given at that point.)

−3   The behaviour of doctor and/or patient shows that honest communication between them has broken down completely. Their relationship, if it can be called one, is marked by insincerity and restriction of communication.

172

RATING OF TENSIONS AROUND THE PATIENT

This refers to the patient's life situation: the tension between the patients and the significant people around him. (The rating of this category also takes into account the overall state of health of these significant others, and their relationships, in as much as they are seen to be affected by the patient's condition).

+3 Mutually satisfactory relationships prevail between the patient and those around him.

+2 Fairly satisfactory relationships exist between the patient and those around him.

+1 Tolerable relationships exist between the patient and those around him.

  0 There is little or no positive quality in the relationships between the patient and those around him.

−1 Relationships between the patient and those around him are fairly strained and troubled.

−2 Relationships between the patient and those around him are marked by trouble and conflict.

−3 Relationships between the patient and those around him have broken down completely as a result of trouble and conflict.

RATING OF THE INTERMEDIATE THERAPEUTIC OBJECTIVE (I.T.O.)

+3 I.T.O. achieved as stated.

+2 Considerable work done with respect to the I.T.O.

+1 Some work done with respect to the I.T.O.

  0 Little or no work done with respect to the I.T.O.

−1 Work done in some opposition to the I.T.O.

−2 Work done in considerable opposition to the I.T.O.

−3 Work done in extreme opposition to the I.T.O.

The assignment of ratings appeared at first to be a simple task. In fact, the procedure carried with it a number of problems, some of which were, initially, hidden, and which needed to be resolved.

It was obviously important that follow-up material was always scored with reference to the same base line, by each member of the team. Although this principle appears to be an easy one to observe, it turned out in fact to be very difficult. There seemed to be a natural tendency to fluctuate between assigning scores on the basis of the rating given at the previous follow-up and assigning scores on the basis of the initial ratings. When this was discovered it was decided that, apart from the category 'Rating of the Patient's Symptoms', all material would be rated on an absolute basis, i.e. in accordance with the scale as it was laid and not in comparison with previous ratings. In this way, the progress of a patient could be followed, with respect to the rating scales, as on a graph.

However, with regard to evaluation in the category 'Rating of the Patient's Symptoms' it soon became evident that an evaluation could not be carried out except on a relative basis, and it was agreed that the base line for comparison at follow-up would be the state of the patient's symptomatology when last reported on.

There was then the knotty question as to whether 'ideal' or 'reasonable' standards should be used. When using a measuring instrument which is to comprise criteria for evaluating the quality of human life, perhaps the main scource of its unreliability will be the inevitable differences of opinion—again, often hidden and often fluctuating—amongst the assessors. This problem is further complicated by the question as to whether, in considering 'ideal' or 'reasonable' as the standard, we are rating with reference to the patient, his doctor, or to the product of the two in their work together. These problems were never entirely resolved but we attempted to deal with them in the following ways:

1. By specifying and describing, as far as possible, each point on a seven point scale.
2. By carefully discussing and stating the bases and rationale for our ratings prior to the assigning of any scores.*

* The score which was finally allotted in each category for each case was the one held by the majority of the research participants.

174

3. By watching carefully, and correcting for, any inconsistency in the standard used for any particular case.

In effect, the final versions of the scales themselves represent the result of considerable trial and revision, and there was a high degree of—at least internal—reliability amongst the raters in the group in their use; i.e. the meaning of the criteria was clear to, and agreed upon by, the raters and the criteria were used according to these meanings with a high degree of consistency.

Bibliography

Bacal, H.: *Training in Psychological Medicine: An Attempt to Assess Tavistock Clinic Seminars*, Psychiatry in Medicine, 2, 13–22, 1971.

Balint, E.: *The Possibilities of Patient-Centred Medicine*, Journal of Royal College of General Practitioners, **17**, 269, 1969.

Balint, M., Balint, E.: *Psychotherapeutic Techniques in Medicine*, Mind & Medicine Monographs, Tavistock Publications, London, 1961.

Balint, M., Balint, E., Gosling, R., & Hildebrand, P.: *A Study of Doctors—Mutual Selection and the evaluation of results in a training programme for family doctors*, Mind & Medicine Monographs, Tavistock Publications, 1966.

Balint, M.: *The Doctor, His Patient and the Illness*, 1957, revised 2nd ed. Pitman Paperbacks, 1968.

Balint, M., Ornstein. P. H., Balint, E.: *Focal Psychotherapy—An Example of Applied Psychoanalysis*, Mind & Medicine Monographs, Tavistock Publications, 1972.

Bourne, S.: *Referrals made by G.P.s reported in Tavistock Clinic Seminars* (paper at Conference on Seminar Teaching), 1971.

Boyle, C. M.: *The difference between patients' and doctors' interpretations of common medical terms*, Brit. med J., **2**, 286.

Clyne, M. B.: *Night Calls: A Study in General Practice*, Mind & Medicine Monographs, Tavistock Publications, 1961.

Courtenay, M. J. F.: *Sexual Discord in Marriage*, Mind & Medicine Monographs, Tavistock Publications, 1968.

176

Friedman, L. J.: *Virgin Wives,* Mind & Medicine Monographs, Tavistock Publications, 1962.

Greco, R. S.: *One Man's Practice,* Mind & Medicine Monographs, Tavistock Publications, 1966.

Hopkins, P. (Ed.): *Patient-Centred Medicine,* (First International Conference of the Balint Society), Regional Doctor Publications Ltd, London, 1972.

Lancet, Leader, *i,* 35, 1969.

Lask, A.: *Asthma,* Mind & Medicine Monographs, Tavistock Publications, 1966.

Malan, D. H.: *A Study of Brief Psychotherapy,* Mind & Medicine Monographs, Tavistock Publications, 1963.

Menninger, K.: Annals of Internal Medicine, **29,** 318–325, 1948.

Paul, Hugh: *Time and numbers in general practice,* Medical World, **77,** 259, 1952.

Spence, J.: *The Need for Understanding the Individual as part of the Training & Function of Doctors & Nurses,* NAMH 1949. (Reprinted in: *The Purpose & Practice of Medicine,* OUP, London, 1960.)

Index